MEDICATIONS FOR SCHOOL-AGE CHILDREN

The Guilford School Practitioner Series

EDITORS

STEPHEN N. ELLIOTT, PhD
University of Wisconsin–Madison

JOSEPH C. WITT, PhD
Louisiana State University, Baton Rouge

Recent Volumes

Medications for School-Age Children

EFFECTS ON LEARNING AND BEHAVIOR

♦♦♦

Ronald T. Brown
Michael G. Sawyer

Foreword by Martin T. Stein

♦

THE GUILFORD PRESS
New York   London

© 1998 The Guilford Press
A Division of Guilford Publications, Inc.
72 Spring Street, New York, NY 10012
http://www.guilford.com

Printed in the United States of America

This book is printed on acid-free paper.

Last digit is print number: 9 8 7 6 5 4 3 2

Library of Congress Cataloging-in-Publication Data

Brown, Ronald T.
    Medications for school-age children: effects on learning and behavior /
Ronald T. Brown, Michael G. Sawyer; foreword by Martin T. Stein.
        p.   cm. — (The Guilford school practitioner series)
    Includes bibliographical references and index.
    ISBN 1-57230-316-6
    1. Pediatric pharmacology.   2. School nursing.   3. Drugs—
Administration.   I. Sawyer, Michael G.   II. Title.   III. Series.
RJ560.B76   1998
615'.1'083—dc21   97-50080
                                                     CIP

Acknowledgments

◆

This book was written with the assistance and kind support of a number of individuals. As in the past, Martha Hagen's typing and editorial support were exceptional. We are also indebted to the efforts of Joan Donegan, Katie Baer, and Emily Smith for their efforts in editorial assistance and the various clerical aspects related to the preparation of this book. We also are indebted to Sharon Panulla of The Guilford Press for her kind support throughout the various stages of the book's preparation. Moreover, the book would have not reached fruition without the support and encouragement of a number of mentors and collaborators with whom we have conducted our research over the years. Both of us also very much appreciated and benefited from the stimulation of our students and trainees, which significantly enriched our careers over the years. The encouragement and support from our families, who have tolerated missed evenings and weekends, will forever be appreciated. Finally, much of what we have learned in pediatric psychopharmacology has been from the many children and families with whom we have worked over the past several decades. We hope and anticipate that the result of our book will be to advocate for additional funding and research in pediatric psychopharmacology to provide more effective help for children and adolescents with learning and behavioral problems and their families.

Foreword

♦

Recognition and treatment of school-age children with behavioral disorders that affect critical aspects of a child's development has expanded enormously in the last quarter of the 20th century. A number of converging areas of science have interacted with sociocultural changes to produce challenges for child health professionals and educators. Clinicians who work with children are now able to classify behavioral patterns into clusters that have implications for specific therapeutic interventions. Knowledge about the interactions between behavior and learning disabilities has expanded to the point that a comprehensive evaluation of a child with school underachievement is not complete without an assessment of the child's behavior in multiple settings as well as an understanding of strengths and weakness in a variety of educational domains. Standardized psychometric testing is now widely available to assess each child. In addition, increasing expectations for educational achievement have come from parents and a society where employment has become more technologically dependent. Finally, advances in neuroscience have brought about a clearer understanding of the biological foundations of behavior and learning. These scientific advances have fueled the discovery and application of pharmaceutical agents for the treatment of children with behavioral disorders.

How have these trends affected the school-age child? In a society that places a premium on the education of its youth, educational opportunities have been designed to maximize the potential growth and development of each individual child. We no longer accept a high dropout rate among children described as "lazy." These children are now evaluated for a learning disability, a medical disorder, a problem with attention, and for psychological problems inherent in the child or family. Children with disruptive behaviors in the classroom, on the playground, or at home receive an equally comprehensive evaluation. As important, children with developmental disabilities such as mental retardation, pervasive developmental delay, and significant physical handicaps now receive educational assessments and treatment plans that are predicated on maximum achievement of educational and psychological goals.

Treatment strategies available to children with behavioral and learning problems include specific educational interventions, training in social learning skills, individual and family psychotherapy (including supportive counseling), and pharmacological interventions. While all of these treatments benefit some children, medications that target specific behaviors that affect learning and social development have been the most extensively studied form of intervention. *Medications for School-Age Children* is a comprehensive review of pediatric and adolescent psychopharmocology that draws from an extensive research literature spanning the past 30 years. It is an extraordinarily useful clinical guide for psychologists and other professionals who work with children, families, and schools.

Drs. Brown and Sawyer correctly point out that child and adolescent psychologists currently play a major role in the evaluation and management of behavioral and learning disorders in school-age children. This book provides them with knowledge about pharmacokinetics (i.e., the physiology of drugs in the human body), specific indications for medication, potential benefits, and drug side effects. The authors review the pharmacology of the major classes of drugs that affect behavior, including both frequently prescribed and less frequently prescribed medicines. Drugs are grouped into the following categories: stimulants, antipsychotics, antidepressants, antiepileptics, and hypnotics/sedatives. The information is current and references to the scientific literature are appropriately documented. The authors include a discussion of standardized behavior scales used in clinical practice as well as in many of the psychopharmacological studies in the medical literature.

Drs. Brown and Sawyer emphasize that a psychopharmacological knowledge base is most useful to clinical child psychologists and school psychologists as an adjunct to their traditional role in evaluation, education, and psychotherapy. I agree with their impression that once medication is prescribed, there are often shortcomings in the quality with which we monitor the effects of the medication on the individual child. They correctly emphasize that the pediatric psychologist is in a unique position to monitor compliance, behavioral change, academic progress, and side effects of drug therapy. What is needed, in my opinion, is a more rigorous method of communication among teachers, parents, mental health professionals, and the primary care physician. Practicing psychologists, who are either school-based or in a community practice with close ties to school personnel, are in a position to provide ongoing evaluation and monitoring of children on medication. In that the brain of a child continues to develop and mature with new synaptic connections and new neuronal patterns and that this maturation process is impacted by the child's environment, it should not be surprising that behavior and learning patterns change with time. Medications that affect the central nervous system add another factor to those changing patterns. With a comprehensive knowledge about psychopharmocolgy, child psychologists can work with schools and other members of the health team to assure more effective treatments and, it is hoped, improved outcomes.

MARTIN T. STEIN, MD
Professor of Pediatrics
University of California, San Diego

Contents

♦

CHAPTER 1

♦♦♦

Overview

♦

For several reasons, it is increasingly important that psychologists who work with children be knowledgeable about the behavioral, cognitive, and physiological effects of psychotropic medication. First, evidence exists that the use of psychotropic medication for children attending school has increased significantly over the past several years. As a result, psychologists increasingly are responsible for the management of children being treated with psychotropic medication. Second, psychotropic medication affects a number of areas of children's school life that extend well beyond the symptoms the medication is intended to target. Third, problems for which psychotropic medication is used are often first identified at school. Thus, the effectiveness of medication to reduce the severity of these problems is best monitored by staff working in school settings. Finally, the adverse effects of medication are frequently evidenced at school.

Psychologists are in a unique position to monitor and evaluate the effects of medication on children's learning and behavior in school settings. The opportunities for observing both the efficacy and the side effects of psychotropic medication are abundant within this context. This is an important issue because, as we highlight throughout this book, much more research is needed to assess both the efficacy and safety of psychotropic medication. Because of their extensive training in research methodology, psychologists need to participate in these research efforts, particularly in studying the effects of medication on learning and behavior within the context of a classroom setting.

Psychologists have specialized expertise in the assessment of children's learning and behavior, as well as the capability of developing and evaluating intervention programs that can assist children in managing the issues and problems associated with school-related difficulties (R. T. Brown, Lee, & Donegan, in press). However, if they are to effectively participate in these research endeavors, psychologists must be familiar with the fundamental aspects of psychotropics, including indications for use, potential benefits, and adverse side effects. As Forness and Kavale (1988) indicated, school personnel also must be able to communicate effectively with health care providers, assist in the selection of appropriate medication to manage specific symptoms, adjust of doses of medication, and document adverse side effects. The importance of these issues is underscored in recent surveys showing that the majority of school and clinical child psychologists provide services to children who receive some type of psychotropic medication (Barkley, McMurray, Edelbrock, & Robbins, 1990; Kubiszyn & Carlson, 1995).

Over the past several decades, interest in the biology of learning and psychiatric disorders has burgeoned (for review, see R. T. Brown & Donegan, 1995). Significant technological developments in the field of neural sciences spawned an impressive initial research program in the psychopharmacology literature. Strong advancements were made in the field of neurophysiology, especially toward increased understanding of the role of neurotransmitters in human emotions and behaviors. Of particular relevance is research examining the role of learning and memory at the level of the synapse (Shaywitz & Shaywitz, 1994).

The progress of diagnostic and neuroimaging techniques with children and adolescents has permitted a careful and systematic study of the role of the central nervous system (CNS), particularly the brain, in various psychiatric and developmental disorders (R. T. Brown & Donegan, 1995). To aid in understanding the interface of any pathology of the CNS with cognition, behavior, and brain functioning, an armamentarium of increasingly sophisticated measures has been developed for both research and clinical use. One example of this technology is the positron emission tomography (PET) scan. A PET scan is a radiographic technique that produces cross-sectional images of the brain from which positively charged particles (positrons) are measured from multiple directions (Ayd, 1995). After recording these measurements, a computer program determines the amount of radioactivity from each point within the brain. Zametkin, Nordahl, and Gross (1990) successfully employed PET scans in their program of research. The data from PET scans of their subjects allowed the researchers to identify the role of the frontal lobe in the brains of young adults with a history of attention-deficit/hyperactivity disorder (ADHD).

The past decade is frequently referred to as the age of the brain. In pediatric populations, significantly increased understanding has occurred in such areas as the influence of hormones in various psychiatric and learning disorders, the influential roles of neurotransmitters, and the structural differences in the brains of children with learning disabilities and/or various psychopathologies compared to those of their normally developing peers. With the advancement of neuroradiological and electrophysiological assessment techniques, a more complete understanding of the CNS and its role in cognitive processes in general, and in learning and mental disorders specifically, is now possible.

INCREASED PREVALENCE OF MEDICATION

The increasing use of psychopharmacology to treat childhood emotional and behavioral disorders means that professionals responsible for the care of children with these disorders must be knowledgeable about the effects of psychotropic drugs. Compelling data show an increase in the use of psychotropic medication for schoolchildren. Gadow (1993b) noted that the initial rationale for determining the extent of medication used to manage child and adolescent psychiatric and learning disorders was to identify possible overdiagnosis and resulting overtreatment with medications. For example, in a major metropolitan area in the southeastern United States, the media alleged (Perl, 1992) that Ritalin (methylphenidate), one of the stimulant medications typically used for the management of ADHD, was being overprescribed to schoolchildren. Reports further suggested that the medication was being used to enhance achievement even in undiagnosed children. Table 1.1 presents the data from these reports, showing the prevalence of Ritalin use by Zip code. Data indicate that the highest amount of use is in the northern suburbs of a major metropolitan area, a higher socioeconomic region of the southeast. This suggests that more af-

TABLE 1.1. Prevalence of Ritalin Use in the Southeast

Metro areas	Zip code clusters	Grams prescribed
Atlanta suburbs	300	11,950
Birmingham	352	10,067
Virginia suburbs of Washington, D.C.	220	6,256
Miami suburbs	331	5,790
Louisville suburbs	402	5,523
Memphis	381	5,165
Charlotte	282	5,020
New Orleans suburbs	700	3,097

Note. From R. Perl (1992). Reprinted by permission from *The Atlanta Journal* and *The Atlanta Constitution.*

fluent families may have access to continuing medication not necessarily available to children from less affluent families.

As Gadow (1993b) pointed out, data pertaining to "pattern of treatment" (i.e., the frequency with which medications are prescribed, dosage and schedule, polypharmacy, age at onset, and duration of treatment) are difficult to ascertain. Reasons include the ambiguities associated with psychiatric diagnoses, the nonspecificity of drug effects that are connected with some psychotropic medications, the difficulty in gathering information pertaining to the use of psychotropic medication to individuals within a particular community, and the lack of a standard for assessing the overuse of medications.

Gadow (1993b) suggested that treatment surveys in the area of psychopharmacology, particularly compared to investigations examining treatment efficacy and safety, have low scientific status, which tends to decrease publication of findings, resulting in a dearth of studies pertaining to prevalence and pattern of these drug treatments for learning and psychiatric disorders in children and adolescents. For those few studies that are available, psychosocial variables associated with treatment prevalence were examined because they might predict prescribing practices. Psychosocial variables primarily include demographic data that determine factors for frequency of prescribing. Such variables include race, gender, birth order, and socioeconomic status (SES). In the adult literature, investigators provide data suggesting that individuals from minority groups (e.g., African American or Hispanic) who also come from low-income areas are at greater risk for certain medication-prescribing practices. For example, a diagnosis of schizophrenia is more likely to be made in individuals from lower SES backgrounds than is a diagnosis of bipolar (manic depressive) disorder. As a result, specific types of medications used to manage symptoms associated with schizophrenia (i.e., antipsychotics) tend to be employed more frequently for individuals from lower SES groups than for their more affluent counterparts.

Patterns of treatment have been most extensively studied for children and adolescents with developmental disabilities and those diagnosed with externalizing behavior disorders (e.g., ADHD). Comorbidity of ADHD with learning disabilities and other developmental disabilities, including mental retardation, is common. Not surprisingly, the prevalence of pharmacotherapy among children in special education programs is quite high, ranging from 6% to 26% (Gadow, 1993b). Prevalence rates for pharmacotherapy are highest in self-contained classrooms for pupils with learning disabilities (25%) and range from 13% to 17% for children receiving special education services for mental retardation. Fewer data are available for children and adolescents who were diagnosed with internalizing disorders (e.g., anxiety disorders, and depression).

Disruptive Behavior Disorders

The majority of surveys of pediatric psychotropic drug use involving the disruptive behavior disorders focus on children suffering from ADHD. Fewer surveys of psychotropic drug use are available on medication management of conduct disorders and oppositional defiant disorder (for review, see, R. T. Brown et al., in press).

Relative to children with other disruptive behavior disorders (i.e., conduct disorder and oppositional defiant disorder), the lay community has shown significant interest in the number of prescriptions of stimulant medication written for schoolchildren believed to be suffering from ADHD. Much of this interest has stemmed from the premise that stimulant medication is sometimes used unnecessarily and even capriciously as a substitute for appropriate teacher–pupil ratios and special education services (Gadow, 1993b). With regard to treatment prevalence, earlier studies generally suggested a use rate of 1–2%, with stimulant medication being most frequently prescribed (Gadow, 1993b). Significant variability in prescribing practices was noted, with the rates of prescribing being more frequent for children from more affluent homes and for younger children attending the public schools, which have fewer self-contained special education classrooms.

Anecdotal evidence suggested that children from either minority groups or low SES backgrounds were more likely to receive medication for the management of externalizing behavioral disorders, including stimulant medication for ADHD (Gadow, 1993b). However, systematic surveys do not support this view and instead suggest that psychopharmacological approaches are employed less frequently for children from lower SES homes than for those children from more affluent backgrounds. The relationship between SES background and use of medication was revealed to be complex.

Safer and Krager (1988, 1989) conducted biannual community surveys in Baltimore County, Maryland, of stimulant medication use for the management of ADHD in the school setting. The data revealed that the prevalence of treatment doubled every 4–7 years and that 2.8% of the school population received medication during 1996 (Safer, Zito, & Pine, 1996). This number reflected an increase of about 250% in the use of stimulant medication from 1990, but a smaller increase than some predicted. Safer et al. (1996) attributed the increased use of stimulants partly to the improved image of the medication and partly to the fact that children were being managed with stimulants for longer periods.

Interestingly, rates of stimulant drug use were found to be highest for 8- and 9-year-olds and lowest for high school students; in all cases, males were managed more frequently with stimulants than were females, with the ratio being 5:1 in favor of males (Safer & Krager, 1988, 1989; Safer et al., 1996). Children attending public schools were more likely to be treated with stimulants for ADHD relative to their peers who attended private schools. Pediatricians were found to be the physicians who most frequently prescribed stimulants to schoolchildren.

Internalizing Disorders

Relative to the disruptive behavior disorders, few studies have investigated prevalence rates of pharmacotherapy for children and adolescents diagnosed with depression, overanxious disorder, or obsessive–compulsive disorder. In large part this is due to the dearth of treatment studies in these populations. Kovacs, Feinberg, Crouse-Novak, Paulauskas, and Finkelstein (1984), in a 5-year longitudinal investigation of 65 children diagnosed with depression, reported that only 2 children in the study were managed with antidepressant medication. Similarly, in a sample of adolescents diagnosed as having major depressive disorder, Keller, Lavori, Beardslee, Wunder, and Ryan (1991) found that only one of the youths received medication, whereas approximately 15% received psychotherapy. Consistent with these findings, Kovacs et al. (1984) reported that only two-thirds of their sample received some type of psychological intervention. No studies were located that examined the prevalence of antianxiety agents in children or adolescents, although one survey of 14 state facilities in New York reported that while nearly 50% of the patients were treated with antipsychotic agents, only 7% were treated with antianxiety agents (Gadow, 1993b).

Developmental Disabilities

The prevalence of medication use was studied for children and adults with developmental disabilities in institutional settings, community-based facilities, and public schools. Data reveal that lower mental abilities increase the likelihood of psychotropic medication being prescribed (Gadow, 1993b).

Mental Retardation

Researchers estimate that 30–60% of individuals with mental retardation were managed with the use of psychotropic medications (Gadow, 1993b). In large part, litigation related to the mistreatment of the mentally retarded in residential facilities drives surveys pertaining to rates of pharmacotherapy for these individuals. Hill and associates (Hill, Balow, &

Bruininks, 1985; Hauber, Bruininks, Hill, & Lakin, 1984) extensively studied psychopharmacology practices affecting children and adolescents in residential and community-based facilities. Up to one-third of individuals who were moderately, severely, or profoundly retarded were receiving some type of psychotropic medication, with the majority receiving antipsychotic drugs. Some individuals also were receiving stimulant medication. In recent years, an increased effort has been made to reduce both the number and dosages of psychotropic medications that these individuals receive (Gadow, 1993b).

Approximately 5% of children and adolescents with trainable mental retardation who are able to attend school programs receive medication for the management of their behavior (Gadow, 1993b). Most receive stimulant medication, and smaller numbers receive antipsychotic and antiepileptic medication. For children and adolescents designated as educable mentally retarded, Cullinan, Gadow, and Epstein (1987) found that up to 15% of the children were receiving psychotropic medication for behavior disorders. Of these medications, stimulants accounted for about one half and antipsychotic medications accounted for another one third.

Autism

In contrast to many other psychiatric disorders and developmental disabilities, there is a low incidence of autism among schoolchildren. Nonetheless, it remains a severe disorder in which psychotropic medication is often used to reduce severe symptoms. Archival information from the Institute for Child Behavior Research in San Diego show rates of pharmacotherapy for children diagnosed with this disorder. Rimland (1988) analyzed parents' perceptions of efficacy pertaining to psychotropic medication for more than 4,000 children. Those agents most frequently used to manage the symptoms associated with autism included the antipsychotic medications (i.e., thioridazine and chlorpromazine), fenfluramine, stimulant medication, and diphenhydramine (Benadryl). The antipsychotic agents and fenfluramine were endorsed by parents as being most effective, and the stimulants were rated as least effective.

Neurological Disorders

Those neurological disorders surveyed with regard to the prevalence of psychotropic medication use include the seizure disorders and Tourette's disorder. It is important for psychologists to be familiar with the effects of antiepileptic medications on cognition and learning. Antipsychotic agents are also frequently used to manage Tourette's disorder.

Seizure Disorders

Reports indicate that there are 150,000–324,000 cases of epilepsy in the United States (for review, see Gadow, 1993b). Because seizure disorders occur at a higher frequency for those who have sustained some compromise of brain function (either prenatal, postnatal, or congenital), there is a higher frequency of antiepileptic drug therapy for individuals with such developmental disabilities as mental retardation, autism, and cerebral palsy. For example, estimates indicate that up to one third of children and adolescents diagnosed with autism received antiepileptic medication for seizures during some period in their lives, with the incidence of seizure disorders being highest during early childhood and again in adolescence (Deykin & MacMahon, 1979; Gillberg, 1991; Volkmar & Nelson, 1990).

It is estimated that between 0.4% and 1.0% of children in the United States have some type of active seizure disorder requiring management with an antiepileptic medication (Hauser & Hesdorffer, 1990), with the highest number being under the age of 2 years (Gadow, 1993b). Reports also suggest that some children are administered antiepileptic medication for periods longer than necessary (Emerson, et al., 1981; Holowach, Thurstone, & O'Leary, 1972; Todt, 1984). In part, this is attributed to the lack of specific procedures for assessing drug response (Gadow, 1993b).

Approximately one-third of persons with mental retardation who were institutionalized, both in this country and in other English-speaking countries, receive medications for seizure disorders (Aman & Singh, 1988; Gadow & Poling, 1988). Gadow (1993b) also observed that for many of these individuals, the use of medication may be prolonged unnecessarily. The incidence of such medication use in institutions for individuals with developmental disabilities ranges from 15% to 20% (Aman & Singh, 1988; Gadow & Poling, 1988). Frequently, separate medications for seizure disorders and externalizing behavior disorders are administered, with each medication having its own unique adverse effects (Aman, Field, & Bridgman, 1985; Gadow & Kalachnik, 1981).

Tourette's Disorder

Stefl, Bornstein, and Hammond (1988) reported on a survey of individuals with Tourette's disorder who were residing in Ohio. Only 43% were receiving active medication at the time of the survey, although 71% of the sample reported receiving medication for Tourette's at some time in their life. Some individuals received clonidine, but the most commonly used pharmacotherapy agent was haloperidol (an antipsychotic agent). Haloperidol was reported by the patients to produce the most symptomatic relief. Over one half of the sample reported they were prescribed stimulant medication, and the majority noted that this class of psychotropics actually made tic symptoms worse. Gadow (1993b) noted that the high degree of dissatisfaction with drug therapy among individuals with Tourette's can be attributed to the high frequency of adverse side effects associated with the psychotropic medications frequently used for Tourette's.

Summary

Most surveys pertaining to the prevalence of psychotropic medications have been conducted on children diagnosed with ADHD and mental retardation. The stimulants are prescribed most frequently for those children diagnosed as ADHD by pediatricians. Use of stimulant medication increased over the years, and estimates indicate that approximately 3% of schoolchildren in the United States currently receive stimulant medication for the management of ADHD. Most children are treated during the elementary school years, although an increasing number of children are being maintained on medication for longer periods.

Antipsychotic medications are frequently employed to manage the problems of children with mental retardation. For children with seizure disorders, antiepileptic medications are most commonly prescribed, although there are few criteria against which to measure the effectiveness of these medications when used with children. Finally, few data available pertain to the frequency of prescribing practices for depression and anxiety disorders.

Gadow (1993b) has suggested that psychotropic medications are overprescribed, considering the base rates of target symptoms for specific disorders and the availability of psychotherapies and psychoeducational programs for many psychiatric disorders found in children and adolescents. Further, few practitioners actually make use of assessment measures that are available for the monitoring of drug response. In addition, most physicians prefer pharmacotherapy to psychological interventions (Gadow, 1993b). Finally, there are a number of psychotropic medications being prescribed that either have not been approved for use with children and adolescents or for which no empirical data are available to guide safety and efficacy.

SOCIAL-ECOLOGICAL PERSPECTIVE

Psychotropic medications affect a number of areas of children's lives that extend well beyond the symptoms for which the medications are intended. For this reason, administration of psychotropic medication must consider the effects of these medications on the broader lives of children and adolescents and on significant others in their environment. For example, although the effectiveness of stimulant medication to reduce the symptoms of ADHD is consistently demonstrated across numerous studies (R. T. Brown et al., in press), questions remain regarding the impact of medication regimens on children's broader social environments. As Whalen, Henker, and Dotemoto (1981) astutely observed, a treatment that has the potential to produce significant behavioral changes in children should concomitantly produce changes in those who interact with these children. Thus, the far-reaching social ramifications of medication deserve consideration. Psychotropic medications influence not only the children for whom they are prescribed but also parents, teachers, and peers with whom these children interact.

Parents

Medications prescribed to children can have a significant impact on maternal–child interaction patterns. For example, mothers with sons in whom ADHD was diagnosed were found to treat their sons in ways that are less controlling, less intrusive, less critical, more positive, and warmer when the sons were receiving active stimulant medication instead of placebos (Barkley & Cunningham, 1979; C. E. Cunningham & Barkley, 1979; Humphries, Kinsbourne, & Swanson, 1978; Schachar, Taylor, Wieselberg, Thorley, & Rutter, 1987).

Teachers

In a systematic program of research, Whalen and Henker and associates hypothesized that medication may alter particular transactions within the classroom, including teacher behaviors (for review, see Whalen & Henker, 1991a). In one of the earliest investigations of this issue, Whalen, Henker, and Finck (1981) showed that when boys with ADHD received placebos, their names were called more frequently than when the same boys were receiving active medication.

An investigation of medication effects by Whalen and associates compared classroom situations that differed according to stimulation (i.e., noisy vs. quiet) and source of regulation (self-paced vs. other-paced) (Whalen, et al., 1978; Whalen, Henker, Collins, Finck, & Dotemoto, 1979). An intriguing medication-by-situation interaction emerged whereby boys receiving placebos versus active medication were readily distinguishable from their peers only in the noisy condition. Boys in whom ADHD was diagnosed were perceived as more intense (defined as behavior that showed high expenditure of energy) when receiving placebos than when taking active medication, but only under other-paced conditions (when they could not regulate their own activities). During the self-paced periods, intensity was perceived as lower and independent of medication status. These findings underscore the contention that medication may interact with the classroom ecology to produce significant behavioral improvements in children.

In a summer school program involving children diagnosed with ADHD, Whalen, Henker, and Dotemoto (1980, 1981) observed teacher interactions with these boys as well as with same gender peers who had not received this diagnosis during classroom activities. A double-blind medication–placebo design was employed in which the boys received either placebos or active medication. The teachers were unaware of the children's diagnosis or whether the children were receiving active medication or placebo. Findings revealed that the teacher was more intense and controlling toward the boys who had been diagnosed with ADHD and who were receiving placebos than toward either the boys with ADHD who were medicated or the normally developing comparison controls. The teachers' behavior did not differ between the subjects with ADHD who were medicated and the controls who were neither diagnosed with ADHD nor medicated. In the midst of engaging in everyday classroom activities, teachers were quite responsive to the medication status of the pupils.

These findings have significant implications for the social-ecological effects of medicating schoolchildren. As Whalen, et al. (1980) observed, "medication may redirect the ongoing streams of transactions in the classroom" (p. 1282). Moreover, alterations in teacher behaviors may have an impact on other children by virtue of the teacher's reallocation of attention, thereby providing greater reinforcement to peers (Whalen, Henker, & Dotemoto, 1981).

Peers

Given the well-documented effects of medication on adult reactions and perceptions, it seems likely that medication use may also affect classmate and peer behaviors. In one of the earliest studies addressing this issue, Whalen, Henker, Collins, McAuliffe, and Vaux (1979) examined communication patterns of school-age boys who participated in a communication task. Boys in whom ADHD was diagnosed were administered either stimulant medication or placebos and compared to boys serving as controls. Regardless of medication status, boys with ADHD were less likely than comparison peers to modulate their behavioral patterns in response to externally imposed shifts in role-appropriate behaviors. The boys with ADHD relative to their peers were unable to maintain consistent, uninterrupted goal orientation or to respond to subtle social learning opportunities. Although the perception of peers on the communication competence of children with ADHD was not directly assessed, the study is important because it demonstrates that medication had little impact on the communication competence among youth who were diagnosed with ADHD with their peers.

In a later series of investigations of peer perceptions of medication effects and ADHD, Whalen, Henker, Castro, and Granger (1987) studied peer sensitivity to medication-related behavioral differences in social behaviors between youth with ADHD and their normally developing comparison peers. In the first study, normally developing sixth-graders rated videotapes of boys with and without ADHD who were engaged in a social interaction game. One half of the boys who had been diagnosed with ADHD were receiving active medication, and the other half were receiving placebos. In the second study, fourth- and sixth-graders rated comparison controls and boys with ADHD treated with either active medication or placebos. All boys played the same interaction game. Both studies found that boys with ADHD who were receiving placebos were perceived by peers as exhibiting more externalizing behaviors (i.e., overactivity, noncompliance, and aggression) than were either medicated boys or comparison controls. The data indicated a keen ability by peers to detect treatment-related differences in the social behaviors of their classmates.

In a summer enrichment research program at the University of California at Los Angeles, Whalen, Henker, Castro, and Granger (1987) compared peer appraisals of boys who had been diagnosed with ADHD following administration of both active medication and placebos. Medication, particularly at higher doses, was found to enhance social standing and increase nominations of boys with ADHD as best friends, fun to be with, and cooperative. The medication-related improvements, however, did not normalize peer appraisals, and there was significant variability in peer ratings in response to medication.

Finally, Granger, Whalen, and Henker (1993) examined perceptions of medication effects on peer interactions of children with ADHD. College students ($n = 86$) were requested to observe videotapes of two boys with ADHD playing an interaction game with three peers. One boy was receiving active medication; the other was receiving placebo. Interestingly, the boy receiving placebo was rated more negatively for poorly controlled behaviors including noncompliance, aggression, and disruption, whereas the medicated boy obtained negative evaluations for social inhibitions such as passive and submissive behaviors. Although the medication condition did not influence observers' perceptions of positive social behaviors, it did influence the type of negative peer perceptions.

The wealth of data provided by Whalen and associates highlights the effect of medication use on the status of boys with ADHD with peers. As Whalen and Henker (1991a) astutely observed, "peers are powerful brokers of treatment effects" (p. 235), and the influence of medication on classmates' perceptions of their peers is clear. Again, this program of research attests to the social-ecological effects of medication on children, their adult caretakers, and their peers.

Children

There is little doubt that many medications administered to children cause changes in learning and behavior. Of interest are the perceptions of the children themselves regarding these changes. For example, stimulant medication compared to placebo has been shown to result in a greater ability of children with ADHD to recognize and acknowledge angry feelings (Whalen & Henker, 1991a). For many children, medication may come as a welcome relief after years of failure and frustration. In fact, some studies provide compelling data that medication has the powerful effect of enhancing the associations between children's self-evaluations and objective performance levels on cognitive tasks (Hinshaw, Henker, & Whalen, 1984; Milich, Licht, Murphy, & Pelham, 1989). More important, as Whalen and Henker (1991a) have observed, when the child rather than the pill is perceived as the impetus for beneficial effects, positive reactions and expectations ensue and the child's future is viewed more optimistically.

Summary

There is ample evidence that some medications exert significant beneficial effects in children in the areas of learning and behavior, and compelling data suggest that medication has a marked effect on significant others within the child's environment. In short, evidence demonstrates that psychotropic medication exerts significant effects on children's lives that extend well beyond symptoms for which the medication was originally intended. Specifically, evidence confirms a social-ecological effect of medication treatment (Whalen & Henker, 1991a), particularly in the enhancement of the perceptions of children by adult caretakers. Some evidence also suggests changes in peer perceptions of medication-related improvements. Further, the perceptions of the children themselves are of prime importance, especially when children see themselves, rather than the medication, as the impetus for behavioral change. Of the psychotropic medications available for children, the social ecology of the stimulants is the most extensively studied, probably because stimulants are the most prevalent form of pharmacotherapy for psychiatric disorders. No studies were located that focused on the social ecology of other types of psychotropic medication employed for children and adolescents. This area remains potentially fruitful for research.

MONITORING SAFETY AND EFFICACY

As noted earlier, treatment efficacy frequently must be monitored at school because the classroom setting is a key setting where medication exerts changes in behavior and cognition. Moreover, side effects of medication are frequently evidenced at school. Psychologists within the context of the school setting are in a unique position to participate in the monitoring of medication on children's learning and behavior. These are important issues because there is continuing controversy about the use of medication for the management of behavioral problems in classroom settings. This controversy centers around the notions that psychiatric diagnoses, particularly ADHD, are sometimes based on insufficient normative data, that adjustment of dose of medication is not made in a systematic fashion, and that standardized measurements are not used frequently enough to assess drug response.

Many benefits can result from contact between the prescribing physician and the classroom teacher, because parents frequently adjust the dose of medication on their own with little input from the classroom teacher. As Gadow (1993b) pointed out, many concerns within the lay community have in fact been confirmed empirically by the scientific community. This issue frequently resurfaces and has spurred interest within the scientific community to determine how psychologists may best participate in school settings to monitor both the efficacy and the safety of psychotropic medication.

Numerous investigations have revealed that specific drug effects may exert improvement in classroom behavior and enhance a child's attention and concentration so that improved academic performance may occur (for review, see R. T. Brown et al., in press). Conversely, some psychotropic agents in sufficiently high doses compromise learning and inhibit behavior (R. T. Brown, Dingle, & Landau, 1994; R. T. Brown et al., in press). Thus, a careful, continuing, and systematic evaluation of various medications on children's learning and behavior must be a basic component of the medical assessment and treatment. The prescribing physician is obligated to ensure ongoing monitoring of the cognitive and behavioral effects of any psychotropic medication. Psychologists can provide an important clinical and investigative role assisting physicians in assessing the clinical efficacy of medication. They can also play an important role in evaluating the efficacy and safety of various psychotropics. Because large numbers of schoolchildren are being treated with psychotropic medication, it is essential that psychologists be familiar with the basic principles of psychopharmacology. This familiarity will increase their ability to monitor and assess the effects of prescribed medication and assist in the identification and reporting of adverse side effects (Barkley, McMurray, et al., 1990; DuPaul & Kyle, 1995).

A role for psychologists in the delivery of mental and general health services in schools is also emerging (DeMers, 1995; Gutkin, 1995), dictated in part, by a recognition of the key role of school personnel in the delivery of psychological health care to children. This recognition is driven by the dearth of available health care services in outpatient clinics within the public sector and the high cost of health care in both the private and the public sectors. Moreover, an insufficient number of mental health care providers are adequately trained to serve children and adolescents. In response to these issues, C. L. Carlson, Paavola, and Talley (1995) reviewed a model of a "full-service school" in which the provision of mental health services is proposed as a core component of the job description of most school psychologists. In accord with this role of the school psychologist and because pharmacotherapy is now an integral component of the mental health services provided to so many children and adolescents, the institution of training policies for psychologists within this area is a high priority for the next decade.

RESEARCH OPPORTUNITIES

Within the field of child psychiatry and developmental and behavioral pediatrics, there is a significant increase in the use of psychotropic medication. In contrast to adult populations, however, medication used for learning and behavior problems in pediatric populations is typically employed as an adjunct to more traditional educational approaches and psychotherapies, such as special education, behavior management, and family systems therapy. The revolution in pediatric psychopharmacology developed, in part, because of the increasing recognition that many learning and behavior disorders in school-age children have a biological component (R. T. Brown & Donegan, 1995; Kruesi et al., 1990). Indeed, a number of pharmaceutical agents have been developed in recent years that show particular promise in enhancing cognitive functioning and improving behavior in children and adolescents (Gadow, 1992). Despite the very exciting advancements in the neurosciences and in psychopharmacology, however, research pertaining to psychotropic medication for children is progressing at a much slower rate than investigations of these medications involving adults. Moreover, the clinical use of psychotropic medications for children and adolescents has surpassed research knowledge concerning their safety and efficacy. This is a dilemma for physicians who are often under pressure to prescribe psychotropic medications even though the efficacy and safety of these agents have yet to be demonstrated for children (R. T. Brown et al., 1994, in press).

Because of their extensive training in research methodology, psychologists have the potential to be valuable participants in psychopharmacology research efforts, particularly in studying the effects of medication on learning and behavior in classroom settings. Neurobiological research has resulted in the development of pharmacological agents that can target specific anatomical and biochemical anomalies of children with learning and emotional disorders. This program of study is still in its infancy but it holds the promise of many more developments to come. Technological achievements have allowed a more precise understanding of the biological factors believed to mediate developmental and psychiatric disorders. An unfolding of pharmaceutical interventions to manage these disorders has been one result. In fact, the use of medication has become a key treatment modality for the management of a number of psychiatric disorders in adults, supplemented by various psychotherapies (R. T. Brown et al., 1994). In short, the significant developments in the neural sciences have been paralleled by advances in psychopharmacology.

Werry and Aman (1993b) have observed that much of the knowledge of pediatric psychopharmacology directly derives from the principles of adult psychopharmacology. The qualitative and quantitative differences between children and adults mandate greater research efforts with children and adolescents and those individuals with developmental disabilities. Brown and colleagues (R. T. Brown et al., 1994, in press) noted that the school setting provides an ideal, ecologically sound laboratory where research efforts can examine the effects of medication on cognition, learning, and behavior in pediatric populations. Further, there is a natural affinity between the skills emanating from the training of psychologists and the expertise required to conduct research in pediatric psychopharmacology. Psychologists with extensive training in the principles of learning, assessment, and rigorous research methodology are in a prime position both to design and to conduct research studies in this area. Until recently, pediatric psychopharmacology research was primarily descriptive, without a great deal of scientific theory utilized to inform and drive this research. The training and expertise of psychologists can assist all practice and scientific disciplines, contributing to the development of more theoretically driven and sound research models by which to study pediatric psychopharmacology.

FORMAT OF THE BOOK

Seven chapters follow. Chapter 2 presents basic terminology pertaining to psychopharmacology, including pharmacokinetics, tolerance, dependence and addiction, drug interactions, and adverse effects. Chapter 3 reviews the short-term effects of psychotropic medication, with particular emphasis on how these medications affect learning and behavior. Chapter 4 reviews the long-term outcome of psychotropic medications, including the influence of these medications on cognition, academic performance, and physical effects. Chapter 5 describes the clinical use of psychotropic agents. Chapter 6 presents approaches used in the assessment and monitoring of children who receive psychotropic medication, including the monitoring of physical effects and assessment of adverse effects. This chapter presents a range of assessment approaches including a model approach for assessing medication efficacy.

Issues of unique interest to psychologists are those pertaining to treatment acceptability and satisfaction, compliance, ethical, and cultural issues. Chapter 7 addresses a range of topics of particular relevance to psychologists, including legal issues and informed consent. Finally, because psychopharmacology represents a relatively new area of training and research, particularly for applied practice, Chapter 8 focuses on proposed clinical training and research.

CHAPTER 2

◆◆◆

Basic Principles
of Pharmacology

◆

The purpose of this chapter is to provide definitions of key terms and an overview of basic pharmacological terminology and concepts. *Pharmacology* encompasses the broad area of study pertaining to the physical and chemical effects of drugs in the body; the mechanisms of action of these drugs; and the effects of drugs on body chemistry, physiology, and behavior (Poling, Gadow, & Cleary, 1991a). *Drugs* or *medications* refer to chemical agents that affect living processes. Pharmacology consists of a number of subdisciplines, including *neuropharmacology*, or the discipline devoted to study of the effects of drugs on the nervous system (Smith & Darlington, 1996). Neuropharmacology is the subdiscipline of most relevance for psychologists in their efforts to understand the effects of various drugs on learning and behavior.

Psychopharmacology is that subdiscipline of pharmacology that addresses the effects of drugs on psychological processes and behavior (Poling et al., 1991a). *Clinical psychopharmacology* is the subdiscipline of psychopharmacology concerned with the use of drugs to treat any abnormal behavior. Finally, *pediatric psychopharmacology* is the field specifically concerned with the behavioral and cognitive effects of drugs on children and adolescents. This is a particularly important area of study because children and the psychiatric disorders for which they are treated differ significantly from those of adults.

Estimates indicate that there are more than 10,000 prescription drugs available for use by physicians in the United States, and that an additional 100,000 pharmaceutical products can be purchased without a prescription (Gadow, 1986). *Over-the-counter* drugs are pharmaceuticals that consumers can obtain without a prescription. Psychotropic agents are prescribed for altering mood or behavior.

DEVELOPMENT OF PHARMACEUTICAL AGENTS

Although some drugs derive from natural substances, including plants and animals, most pharmaceuticals derive from synthetic substances (Poling et al., 1991a). Each pharmaceutical agent has a chemical name that describes its molecular structure. When a drug is developed for clinical use, it is assigned a United States Adopted Name (USAN), or the *generic* name of the drug. Generic names typically are used in the empirical and clinical literature throughout the world; hence, we use generic names in this book. Pharmaceutical firms also assign *trade names* to drugs, and these trade names are protected by trademark laws. Trade names used by firms to promote their drugs are chosen to be easily remembered and, in many cases, to suggest the therapeutic application of the drug. For example, methylphenidate is the generic name for a widely used stimulant medication, Ritalin, which is used to manage symptoms associated with ADHD.

Drug manufacturers control the right to produce a particular pharmaceutical agent for 17 years. When this period expires, the drug may be manufactured by other pharmaceutical companies that call their product by its generic label or by a different trade name. Such medications manufactured by other pharmaceutical companies are frequently sold at a lower price than the original product, and, for this reason, may be preferred by physicians and parents.

PHARMACOKINETICS

Routes of Administration

Pharmacokinetics is the absorption, distribution, and elimination of drugs in the body, or, more simply, the body's effect on the drug (Smith & Darlington, 1996). *Pharmacodynamics* is the study of drugs and their actions on the body or the response of the body to chemical agents.

The method administration of a drug influences the speed with which a drug begins to act, the duration of its effect, the changes over time (time course), and the extent of the drug response (Smith & Darlington, 1996). Drugs are administered in several different ways. One method is by mouth: The drug is swallowed or placed *sublingually* (under the tongue). Oral administration of medication is convenient. However, the speed of action of drugs administered orally may vary because absorption can be delayed if a patient's stomach is full. In contrast, a drug administered sublingually is quickly absorbed into circulation because it bypasses the gastrointestinal tract and possible absorption problems. This route of administration can be particularly advantageous for children who are experiencing nausea and vomiting.

Rectal administration may be preferred if a patient is experiencing nausea and vomiting (Smith & Darlington, 1996). Medications can also be inhaled. Inhalation allows drugs to enter the bloodstream rapidly through the lungs. Medications used for reactive airway disease (i.e., asthma) are frequently administered using an inhaler.

Many medications are administered by injection under the skin (*subcutaneously*), into muscle (*intramuscularly*), or into a vein (*intravenously*) (Smith & Darlington, 1996). When drugs are administered subcutaneously or intramuscularly, they exert their effects more rapidly than when they are administered orally. Medications administered intravenously enter directly into the bloodstream. Typically, this method achieves the most rapid action. The intravenous route also provides the best control over the concentration of the drug delivered into the blood plasma. When a drug is injected into the muscle, the blood stream generally absorbs it more slowly via capillaries in the muscle tissues (Poling et al., 1991a). Neuroleptics or antipsychotic drugs can be administered intramuscularly, particularly when rapid sedation is desired for a patient experiencing acute psychotic episodes.

Absorption

Psychotropic agents are usually administered orally in tablet or capsule form. Oral forms are the most convenient route of administration and are typically the safest (Smith & Darlington, 1996). After oral administration, the medication is subsequently dissolved in the fluids of the stomach and in the intestine. Ultimately, the drug's molecules pass through the cells that line the wall of the digestive tract and into the capillaries of the veins that extend from the stomach and small intestine to the liver.

Several variables influence the rate of absorption. These include the chemical comprising the drug, the presence of other drugs in the digestive tract, the acidity of the stomach, the presence of illnesses that may result in a more rapid passage of blood through the stomach, and chemicals in foods that are consumed during drug administration (Smith & Darlington, 1996). The form in which the drug is administered also determines the rate of absorption. For example, liquids are absorbed more rapidly than are solids, and manufacturers can alter the thickness of a pill's coating to hasten or slow absorption. For example, Poling et al. (1991a) noted that providing Ritalin in a form that slows absorption (e.g., sustained-release Ritalin) may prolong the effects of this stimulant medication.

Distribution

Once medication is absorbed into the bloodstream it is distributed throughout the body to various sites of action. The properties of the drug agents determine their sites of action and the concentration of drugs in the blood plasma (Gadow, 1986). Some drugs are largely restricted to the circulatory system, whereas others cross into the CNS. The drug molecules pass through the small arteries and then diffuse out of capillaries to come into contact with the neurons in the brain (Smith & Darlington, 1996). Most drugs combine with large protein molecules in the blood, a process referred to as *protein binding*. Protein binding reduces the maximum effect of drugs but also prolongs their effects because the drug molecules are then released over time (Briant, 1978). Many psychotropic medications also are *lipid soluble*. This enables them to combine with fats and pass into and out of the bloodstream more readily than agents that are not lipid soluble.

The movement of drug molecules from the bloodstream into the brain is in part impeded by the glial cells that surround the capillaries of the brain (Poling et al., 1991a). As a result, capillaries of the brain prevent certain molecules from entering and affecting the neurons. This barrier is referred to as the *blood–brain* barrier (Smith & Darlington, 1996).

Biotransformation and Excretion

Most drugs are broken down into metabolites that are water soluble (Smith & Darlington, 1996). This breakdown primarily occurs in the liver, and the resulting metabolites are then excreted through the kidneys. The metabolism of drugs varies among individuals and may also be affected by the presence of other drugs or chemicals in the body. Some drugs, lithium for example, are not metabolized and pass through the body in an unchanged state.

Although the kidneys are the primary organs responsible for excreting drugs and their metabolites from the body, elimination can also occur in feces, in perspiration, and in the milk of nursing mothers (Smith & Darlington, 1996). The rate of excretion is determined by a range of factors, including the age of the patient, drug history, and presence of liver or kidney disease.

The *half-life* of a drug refers to the amount of time it takes for the body to reduce the amount of drug by 50% (Smith & Darlington, 1996). Some drugs have a half-life that is independent of the dose of the drug and its concentration, whereas the speed of elimination of others occurs in proportion to the amount of increase in the dose or concentration of the drug. For drugs that are long-acting and characterized by variable half-lives, blood levels and the overt effects may increase over time. This process, *accumulation*, can make measuring behavioral effects of a particular drug agent difficult (Poling et al., 1991a).

DOSE RESPONSE AND INDIVIDUAL VARIATION

Before marketing any drug, manufacturers collect a great deal of data about the effects of various doses of the drug on bodily functioning in both laboratory animals and humans. At very low doses, drugs may produce no observable effects, whereas at very high doses, drugs may produce harmful or toxic effects (Poling et al., 1991a). All psychotropic drugs have recommended minimum and maximum doses. *Titration* is to the process of adjusting the dose of a drug. For example, when an initial dose of medication is too small to achieve a desired effect, the dose must be gradually increased or titrated to higher levels to achieve the desired effect. To achieve the ideal dose for an individual patient, physicians may administer a small amount of medication, which they titrate until they achieve a desired response or until adverse effects appear. If an adverse effect does occur, clinicians can reduce the dose or discontinue the medication and initiate a different medication. Alternatively, another medication may be employed to control the adverse side effect. For example, when muscular rigidity occurs in response to antipsychotic drug therapy, specific anticholinergic agents such as Artane (trihexyphenidyl) or Cogentin (benztropine mesylate) can be administered.

Medication is typically measured in milligrams (mg), with the dosage for children often being expressed as milligrams per kilogram (mg/kg) of body weight. For adults, recommendations are more commonly described as the milligram of medication to be administered each day. Regular monitoring of the amount of drug in the bloodstream may also be used to guide the appropriate dosage. For example, ongoing dosages of lithium and antiepileptic agents are often based on the concentration of the drug in the blood. This concentration is referred to as *blood levels* and is expressed as *micrograms of drug per milliliter* of blood (Poling et al., 1991a). Most psychotropic medications prescribed to manage learning and behavior typically require careful titration or adjustment to reach the most effective dosage for individual patients. In these circumstances, behavioral and learning indices are employed as the barometer for adjusting the dosage of the medication. Although this process is fairly crude and inexact, the amount of medication needed to produce a desired effect frequently varies among individuals, as does the dose associated with adverse side effects. For this reason, the effective dose of a psychotropic agent often varies, sometimes a great deal, for different individuals (Smith & Darlington, 1996).

TOLERANCE

Tolerance occurs when the ongoing administration of a particular dose of medication no longer has a beneficial or desired effect, or when a higher dose is necessary to produce the same effect of a medication (Smith & Darlington, 1996). Tolerance varies across different medications. *Tachyphylaxis* occurs when tolerance for the therapeutic effect of a medication develops very rapidly or after only a few doses of medication. Fortunately, children develop tolerance rather quickly for many of the adverse effects of psychotropic medications. For example, one of the adverse effects of neuroleptic drug therapy is drowsiness; however, most individuals develop tolerance to this particular adverse side effect. *Behavioral tolerance* is the individual's ability to counteract the behavioral effects of the drug, and *metabolic tolerance* indicates that the drug actually has stimulated the metabolic processes responsible for the breakdown of the drug. Thus, when behavioral or metabolic tolerance occurs, the dose of the drug necessary to attain the desired effect must be larger than the previous doses administered.

DEPENDENCE

When cessation of drug therapy produces physical or psychological effects, this is referred to as *physical dependence* (Smith & Darlington, 1996). Physical dependence of a particular pharmacotherapy may result in an alteration in physiological status, changes in behavior, or an alteration in psychological state or mood. Continuous exposure to a drug results in physiological adaptation, and when the drug is withdrawn, the physiological response may actually be in the opposite direction of what is desired. The *rebound phenomenon* is observed when children discontinue stimulant drug therapy; often their inattentiveness and overactivity appear to exacerbate in response to cessation of the stimulant medication (Poling et al., 1991a). Finally, *psychological dependence* of a drug refers to the ongoing self-administration of a medication. The self-administration of caffeine by millions of Americans is a prime example of psychological dependence. Psychological dependence is not necessarily harmful unless the use of the drug results in physical damage.

ADDICTION

Addiction is a behavioral pattern of drug use characterized by the compulsive and harmful use of a drug and the tendency to relapse once the drug is withdrawn (Jaffee, 1985). A person can be addicted to a drug without necessarily being physically dependent on it. In addition, a person can be physically dependent on a drug and not necessarily addicted to the drug (Poling et al., 1991a).

MECHANISMS OF DRUG ACTION

The means by which drugs exert their effects is their *mechanism of action*. The mechanism of action of most drugs is based on a chemical interaction between a drug and an important component of the body (Smith & Darlington, 1996). Most drugs are believed to produce their effects by combining with cell membranes, enzymes, or other specialized components of cells. Pharmacologically active compounds are considered either structurally specific or structurally nonspecific. *Structural specificity* refers to the extent to which a drug produces an effect by combining with a specific receptor. Structurally nonspecific drugs do not combine with specific receptors but instead exert their influence by penetrating into cells or accumulating in cell membranes.

Receptor theory posits that drugs are selectively active substances that have a particular affinity for specific chemical groups and for particular cells (Smith & Darlington, 1996). According to receptor theory, drugs exert their action by attaching to specialized regions of a cell. *Receptors* are the cellular components with which drugs interact to produce specific effects. *Affinity* is to the propensity of a drug to be found at a particular receptor site, and *efficacy* describes the drug's ability to initiate biological activity. Many psychotropic agents are believed to exert their actions at receptor sites. Receptors in the nerve cell are the parts of a cell to which neurotransmitters bind chemically. Receptors include proteins, nucleic acids, and lipids of cell membranes.

DRUG INTERACTIONS AND
ADVERSE SIDE EFFECTS

Some children receive multiple medications throughout the course of a single day. For example, children or adolescents who are diagnosed with a chronic medical illness may simultaneously be receiving psychotropic medication for a learning or behavioral problem or even a seizure disorder. In fact, Gadow (1986) pointed out that up to 10% of children who are in special education programs receive medication for both behavior and seizure disorders. *Polypharmacy* occurs when two drugs are employed simultaneously to manage the same or different disorders; *multiple-drug therapy* refers to prescribing two or more medications for the same disorder (Poling et al., 1991a). Several psychopharmacologists (Poling et al., 1991a; Werry & Aman, 1993b) have cautioned against the use of multiple-drug therapy unless the medications have different mechanisms of action or the clinical efficacy of the combinations of medication is superior to any single psychotropic medication.

When two medications are administered simultaneously, their effects may be additive, that is, their combined effects equal the sum of the individual effects (Smith & Darlington, 1996). Some drugs, however, may be *supra-additive* or *synergistic,* whereby one particular medication affects the absorption, distribution, biotransformation, or excretion of another drug. This characteristic has the potential to either increase or decrease the efficacy or toxicity of another drug. Thus, the physician must evaluate the potential of any harmful drug interactions when a child is being managed with two or more medications. This situation often is a challenge for the physician who treats children suffering from multiple handicapping conditions and/or developmental disorders with a co-occurring physical disorder.

Nearly every drug has side effects, which are commonly referred to in the pharmacology literature as *adverse effects*. These are unwanted physiological, behavioral, or cognitive effects that are associated with the pharmacological reactions of the medication (Gadow, 1986). In addition, adverse effects also may appear in the form of excessive *therapeutic response;* in such a case, adverse side effects typically are dose related. *Behavioral or cognitive toxicity* occurs when medication interferes with behavior or impedes cognitive functioning (Poling et al., 1991a). For example, antipsychotic medications may result in behavioral toxicities if they lead to excess sedation, whereby individuals encounter difficulties in interacting with other people or in socializing appropriately. Cognitive toxicity is an adverse side effect frequently encountered with antiepileptic medications; these agents may result in depressed cognitive functioning, thereby impeding academic or school performance.

Neurophysiology

Because psychotropic drugs exert their therapeutic effects by affecting the nerve cells in the brain, an understanding of the basic features of the CNS, neuroanatomy, and neurophysiology is necessary. The brain consists of 20 million neurons (Poling et al., 1991a). The *neuron* is the basic unit of the nervous system and consists of four parts: (1) the *cell body* (2) *dendrites,* (3) *axon,* and (4) *axon terminals* (R. T. Brown & Donegan, 1995; R. T. Brown & Morris, 1994). The cell body receives messages from the dendrites and subsequently relays the messages to the next cell body via the axon. The messages relayed by the dendrites and axons are conduced by an elaborate *electrochemical process.* The transmission of nerve impulses between the neurons is referred to as *synaptic transmission.* Gaps known as *synapses* exist between the end of one neuron at the axon terminal and the beginning of the next neuron. Communication across synapses takes place via the release of a chemical from one neuron that relays the message to an adjacent neuron that receives the message (R. T. Brown & Morris, 1994).

Communication across synapses is chemically mediated (R. T. Brown & Morris, 1994). The *neurotransmitter* is a chemical that is released into the synapse and subsequently activates the receptor site. Neurotransmitters produce excitation or inhibition in a postsynaptic cell by altering the permeability of the cell's membrane. Although most neurotransmitters can have either excitatory or inhibitory effects at a given synapse, each neurotransmitter is either *excitatory* or *inhibitory,* not both. The neurotransmitter molecules cross the synaptic cleft, the fluid-filled gap between the neurons. Subsequently, the neurotransmitter interacts with receptors on the membrane of the next neuron.

In recent years, many neurotransmitter substances have been identified. Jacobs (1994) suggested that there may be as many as 100 different neurotransmitters within the CNS, although it has not been determined how many transmitters there are in the nervous system. The best understood neurotransmitter is *acetylcholine* (ACH), which is essential for muscular message transmission and also controls basic involuntary processes such as breathing (Kandel, Schwartz, & Jessell, 1991). *Cholinergic neurons* secrete ACH. Myasthenia gravis, a disease involving muscular weakness and fatiguability, is believed to be caused by a loss of ACH receptors in the muscle fibers.

An additional class of neurotransmitters is the bioamines, or biogenic amines. The catecholamines are bioamines and include *epinephrine* (adrenalin), *norepinephrine* (noradrenalin), and *dopamine* (Kandel et al., 1991). These particular transmitters are involved in various facets of personality, mood, and drive states. *Adrenergic neurons* release catecholamines.

Serotonin, another core transmitter, is believed to suppress arousal and to regulate hunger, temperature, sexual behavior, aggression, mood, and the onset of sleep (Kandel et al., 1991). Other essential transmitters include *GABA* (gamma-aminobutyric acid), an inhibitory transmitter of the CNS, and the endorphins, involved in the inhibition of pain.

Neuropharmacology

Over the past several years, there has been a burgeoning of scientific literature pertaining to the role of neurotransmitters in the understanding of human behavior and emotions. These findings led to extensive research in the area of neuropharmacology (R. T. Brown & Donegan, 1995; R. T. Brown et al., in press; R. T. Brown & Morris, 1994). For example, excessive dopamine was posited to be involved in the development of schizophrenia, and low levels of this substance in the basal ganglia of the brain are believed to play a role in the onset of certain movement disorders, including Parkinson's disease (R. T. Brown & Donegan, 1995; R. T. Brown & Morris, 1994). Suppressed levels of GABA in the motor region of the brain are associated with Huntington's chorea, a serious neurological condition that results in death. Of direct relevance to pediatric psychopharmacology is the recent evidence suggesting that learning and memory occur at the level of the synapse, and this may be partly mediated by neurotransmitters, including dopamine (Shaywitz & Shaywitz, 1994).

Mechanisms of Action

Psychotropic medications can alter the synthesis, storage, or release of specific neurotransmitters (Smith & Darlington, 1996). Some psychotropic drugs interfere with the deactivation of neurotransmitters by means of enzymes or by a process known as reuptake. Reuptake refers to the reabsorption of the neurotransmitter from the synaptic cleft back into the original neuron. This decreases the availability of neurotransmitters at receptor sites. Finally, some medications interact with receptor sites themselves (Poling et al., 1991a).

Psychopathology and Learning

The *dopamine hypothesis* posits that schizophrenia is associated with overactivity at dopamine receptors, as a result of either oversensitivity of the receptors or excessive dopamine levels at the site of the receptors. Research suggests that the antipsychotic or neuroleptic agents exert their effects by blocking dopamine receptors in the brain (Smith & Darlington, 1996). Support for the dopamine hypothesis comes from the observation that amphetamines and other drugs that can elevate dopamine levels may produce a psychosis which resembles schizophrenia and administration of low levels of such drugs may also exacerbate symptoms of schizophrenia.

The *catecholamine hypothesis* posits that depression is the result of a deficiency of norepinephrine whereas mania is believed to be due to an excess of this neurotransmitter. The antidepressant medications are believed to exert their effects by blocking the reuptake of norepinephrine and/or serotonin at the synapses, thereby increasing the availability and actions of these neurotransmitters on excitatory postsynaptic cells (Smith & Darlington, 1996). The efficacy of antidepressant medications on norepinephrine and serotonin supports this theory of depression. The *permissive theory* involves both the neurotransmitters norepinephrine and serotonin and suggests that low serotonin levels produce a vulnerability for an affective disorder. Depression is believed to occur when serotonin and norepinephrine are both low, whereas mania is a function of low serotonin levels and high norepinephrine levels. Finally, the two-disease theory suggests that there are two types of depression, one the result of deficiencies in serotonin and the other the result of low levels of norepinephrine.

CONCLUSIONS

The actions of pharmacological agents are complex. Clinicians must consider many details simultaneously when they prescribe any medication to children and adolescents; this is especially important with psychotropic agents. A thorough understanding of pharmacology and human physiology is necessary for prescribing psychotropic agents. The physician must decide the appropriate route of administration and be knowledgeable about the distribution of the drug throughout the body, and the time course of action of the psychotropic agent. The physician also must carefully evaluate the development of tolerance and dependence, as well as potential drug interactions and adverse side effects.

Although a complete understanding of the complex effects of psychotropic medication on physiological functioning is not currently within the scope of applied practice in psychology, the most important marker of psychotropic drug efficacy in pediatric populations is behavioral and cognitive response. Thus, psychologists have much to contribute to the assessment of drug response. The study of behavioral and cognitive response to psychotropic medication—*behavioral psychopharmacology*—is an area that has recently received one of the largest increases in federal research funding in the field of childhood and learning disorders. Moreover, the use of psychotropic agents revolutionized the management of learning and behavioral disorders, and, for this reason, the remainder of this book focuses primarily the behavioral effects of psychotropic medications.

♦♦♦

Short-Term Cognitive and Behavioral Effects of Psychotropic Medications

♦

This chapter reviews the cognitive and behavioral effects of psychotropic medications commonly prescribed for children and adolescents. These medications include the stimulants, the antipsychotics, the antiepileptics, the antidepressants, and the anxiolytics. The focus of the chapter is on the general effects of the medications rather than on their effectiveness when used to treat childhood or adolescent mental health disorders. Table 3.1 presents an overview of each class of medication, the possible indications of each type of medication, and their adverse effects on cognition and behavior.

STIMULANTS

Stimulant medications are among the most meticulously researched of the psychotropic medications. This section reviews stimulant medications as they affect cognition, learning, academic achievement, behavioral and motoric functioning, socialization, and peer relationships.

Cognitive Functioning

A corpus of research consistently demonstrates the ability of stimulant medication to enhance the performance of children on laboratory tasks of cognitive functioning (R. T. Brown, Dingle, & Dreelin, 1997; R. T. Brown et al., in press; Jacobvitz, Sroufe, Stewart, & Leffert, 1990; Rapport & Kelly, 1991). Results generally suggest that stimulants exert significant positive

TABLE 3.1. Common Pharmacological Agents Administered to Children and Adolescents

Class of drug	Generic name	Trade name	Possible Indications	Possible side effects	Serious side effects	Cognitive/behavioral effects
Antidepressants						
Tricyclics	Imipramine	Tofranil	Enuresis Depression	Sedation Dry mouth Constipation Urinary retention	Cardiac conduction slowing with heart block Decrease in seizure threshold Exacerbation of glaucoma	
	Amitriptyline	Elavil	Enuresis	Blurred vision Cardiac conduction slowing		
	Desipramine	Norpramin	ADHD Depression	Mild tachycardia Elevated blood pressure	Possible sudden death from cardiac failure Cardiac arrhythmias	
	Nortriptyline	Pamelor	ADHD Depression	Weight gain Orthostatic hypotension		
	Clomipramine	Anafranil	Depression Obsessive–compulsive disorder	Dry mouth Somnolence Tremor Dizziness Headache Fatigue	Convulsions Coma Hypothyroidism	
Monoamine oxidase inhibitors	Phenelzine	Nardil	Atypical depression—often with anxiety	Dizziness Headache Drowsiness Weight gain	Death from hypertensive crisis Convulsions Progressive hepatocellular damage Leukopenia	

Selective serotonin reuptake inhibitors	Fluoxetine	Prozac	Depression Obsessive–compulsive disorder	Headache Nausea Nervousness Insomnia Diarrhea	Decreased concentration (rare) Anecdotal reports of decreased memory
	Sertraline	Zoloft	Depression	Nausea Headache Diarrhea Insomnia Dry mouth	Decreased concentration (rare)
	Paroxetine	Paxil	Depression Obsessive–compulsive disorder Panic disorder	Nausea Somnolence Headache Dry mouth Low energy	Confusion (rare)
	Fluvoxamine	Luvox	Obsessive–compulsive disorder	Nausea Headache Somnolence Insomnia Low energy Dry mouth	CNS stimulation (rare)
	Venlafaxine	Effexor	Depression	Nausea Headache Somnolence Dry mouth Dizziness	Confusion (rare)

(continued)

TABLE 3.1. (*continued*)

Class of drug	Generic name	Trade name	Possible Indications	Possible side effects	Serious side effects	Cognitive/behavioral effects
Others	Trazodone	Desyrel	Depression Dizziness Nervousness Dry mouth	Hypertension		
	Bupropion	Wellbutrin	Agitation Dry mouth Headache	Hypertension		
Anxiolytics (antianxiety)						
Benzodiazepines	Diazepam	Valium	Seizures Anxiety disorders Behavior disorders Emotional lability	Sedation Drug dependence	Drug abuse	Diminished cognitive performance Confusion
	Lorazepam	Ativan	Anxiety	Excessive sleepiness Drug dependence	Drug abuse Hypertension	Confusion
	Alprazolam	Xanax	Anxiety Panic disorder	Dizziness Fatigue Impaired coordination Drug dependence		Memory impairment Cognitive disorder
Others	Buspirone	BuSpar	Anxiety	Dizziness Drowsiness		Decreased concentration Confusion
	Clorazepate	Tranxene	Anxiety	Drowsiness Dizziness	Abnormal liver functioning Abnormal kidney functioning Drug dependence	

	Generic	Brand	Indication	Common side effects	Serious side effects	
	Diazepam	Valium	Anxiety	Drowsiness Fatigue Ataxia Nervousness	Neutropenia Jaundice Drug dependence	
Antimanics	Lithium carbonate	Eskalith Lithobid Lithonate	Bipolar disorder Aggression	Gastrointestinal upset Tremor Headache Polyuria/polydipsia	Renal injury Thyroid dysfunction Toxicity Ataxia Leukocytosis	
Antipsychotics Phenothizazines	Chlorpromazine	Thorazine	Acute psychotic states	Sedation Orthostatic hypotension	Tardive dyskinesia Neuroleptic malignant syndrome Elevated liver enzymes	Cognitive blunting
	Thioridazine	Mellaril	Autistic disorder Pervasive developmental disorder	Akathisia, motor restlessness Parkinsonian symptoms Photosensitivity	Agranulocytosis Acute dystonic reactions Seizures Retinopathy Rebound hypertension	Cognitive blunting
	Trifluoperazine	Stelazine	Tourette's disorder Dyskinetic movements	Sedation Hypotension Headache Gastrointestinal upset Anticholinergic effects Insomnia	Depression Cardiac arrhythmias	Cognitive blunting
Others	Haloperidol	Haldol	Psychotic disorder	Insomnia Restlessness Anxiety	Tardive dyskinesia Neuroleptic malignant syndrome	Cognitive blunting

(continued)

TABLE 3.1. (*continued*)

Class of drug	Generic name	Trade name	Possible Indications	Possible side effects	Serious side effects	Cognitive/behavioral effects
					Electrocardiographic changes Leukopenia/leukocytosis Agranulocytosis Impaired liver function	
	Thiothixene	Navane	Psychotic disorder	Tachycardia Drowsiness Syncope	Tardive dyskinesia Neuroleptic malignant syndrome Cerebral edema Leukopenia/leukocytosis	Cognitive blunting
	Molindone	Moban	Psychotic disorder	Drowsiness Tachycardia	Tardive dyskinesia Neuroleptic malignant syndrome	Cognitive blunting
	Loxapine	Loxitane	Psychotic disorder	Nausea	Leukopenia/leukocytosis	Cognitive blunting
	Clozapine	Clozaril	Drug-resistant schizophrenia	Drowsiness Dizziness Headache	Seizures Agranulocytosis Tardive dyskinesia Neuroleptic malignant syndrome	Cognitive blunting
Psychostimulants	Dextroamphetamine	Dexedrine	ADHD	Insomnia Dysphoria	Hypertension Psychotic symptoms	Behavioral rebound
	Methylphenidate	Ritalin	ADHD	Anorexia Weight loss or failure to gain	Growth retardation Motor tics	Impaired cognitive performance

	Pemoline	Cylert	ADHD	Weight loss or failure to gain	Liver dysfunction	
	Dextroamphetamine sachharate/ sulfate	Adderall	ADHD	Palpitations Hypertension Exacerbation of tics Restlessness	Cardiomyopathy	
Antihistamines	Diphenhydramine	Benadryl	Anxiety Insomnia	Oversedation Agitation		
	Hydroxyzine	Atarax	Sleep induction Agitation	Incoordination Abdominal pain Blurred vision		
Beta-adrenergic blockers	Propranolol	Inderal	Aggression	Dry mouth		
Anticonvulsants	Phenobarbital	Bellergal-S Donnatal Mudrane	Seizures	Hyperactivity		
	Diphenylhydantoin	Dilantin	Seizures	Irritability Aggression Depressed mood		Memory and attention disturbance
	Carbamazepine	Tegretol	Seizures Aggression	Drowsiness Nausea Irritability Agitation	Bone marrow effects Mania	

(continued)

TABLE 3.1. *(continued)*

Class of drug	Generic name	Trade name	Possible Indications	Possible side effects	Serious side effects	Cognitive/behavioral effects
	Valproic acid	Dapakene Dapakote	Mania Seizures	Nausea Gastrointestinal distress Weight gain Tremor		
	Phenytoin	Dilantin	Seizures	Nystagmus Ataxia Dizziness Insomnia		Confusion
Benzodiazepines	Clonazepam	Klonopin	Seizures	Drowsiness Ataxia	Drug dependence	Confusion
Other drugs	Clonidine	Catapres	Tourette's disorder ADHD Aggression	Sedation Dry mouth Dizziness		
	Naltrexone	Revia	Alcohol dependence	Nausea	Hepatocellular injury at high doses	

effects on tasks that require vigilance and sustained attention (Klorman, Brumaghim, Fitzpatrick, & Borgstedt, 1990; Rapport, Carlson, Kelly, & Petaki, 1993; Rapport & Kelly, 1991), matching-to-sample tasks or measures of inhibitory control (R. T. Brown, Jaffe, McGee, & Silverstein, 1992; R. T. Brown & Sleator, 1979; Douglas, Barr, Amin, O'Neill, & Britton, 1988; Malone & Swanson, 1993; Rapport et al., 1993; Rapport & Kelly, 1991; Tannock, Schachar, Carr, & Logan, 1989; Vyse & Rapport, 1989), more efficient search strategies (Klorman et al., 1990), improved performance on stimulus–reaction time tasks (Douglas et al., 1988; Tannock et al., 1989), enhanced performance on long- and short-term recall tasks (Dalby, Kinsbourne, & Swanson, 1989; Douglas et al., 1988; Evans, Gualtieri, & Amara, 1986; Rapport, Quinn, DuPaul, Quinn, & Kelly, 1989), paired associate learning (Dalby et al., 1989; Douglas et al., 1988; Rapport et al., 1989), picture recognition tasks (Kupietz, Winsberg, Richardson, Maitinsky, & Mendell, 1988; Peloquin & Klorman, 1986; Reid & Borkowski, 1984; Sprague & Sleator, 1977), stimulus identification tasks with and without distraction (Reid & Borkowski, 1984; Sebrechts et al., 1986), and improvement on tasks related to perceptual and motoric functioning (Douglas et al., 1988; Gittelman, Klein, & Feingold, 1983).

Given the beneficial effects of stimulant medication on basic cognitive tasks associated with attention and impulsivity, interest in examining the actions of stimulants on higher-order cognitive tasks is growing (Spencer et al., 1996). For example, Keith and Engineer (1991) demonstrated that methylphenidate enhanced receptive language capacity and auditory processing skills in children diagnosed with ADHD. Although these data are encouraging, the research was conducted in absence of a double-blind trial, rendering replication necessary before definitive conclusions can be accepted about the effects of stimulants on language. Similarly, Malone, Kershner, and Seigel (1988), in their investigation of language processing, found that methylphenidate enhances phonological levels of word processing. They concluded that the therapeutic effects of the stimulants are produced through the inhibition of excessive right-hemisphere activity in response to task demands that activate the left hemisphere. Similarly, Balthazor, Wagner, and Pelham (1991) demonstrated that methylphenidate improves nonspecific aspects of information processing. Thus, although stimulant medication has a significant effect on vigilance, impulse control, fine-motor coordination, and reaction time (for review, see Barkley, DuPaul, & Costello, 1993), Werry (1978) noted that stimulant drugs are unlikely to alter children's capacity to solve higher-order problems.

Several investigations used the paired associates learning task, in which a child is presented with word pairs and subsequently requested to respond with the initial stimulus. Rapport et al. (1989) demonstrated that methylphenidate facilitated acquisition and accuracy on a task of paired associate learning. Specifically, the investigators found that rates of acquisition and accuracy varied with dose of stimulant medication and exposure to the material presented. Methylphenidate enhanced accuracy, and speed of acquisition improved with prior experience to the task. This study is important because it suggests that stimulant medication exerts an influence on specific cognitive processes and that other cognitions may not be affected. Similarly, Sallee, Stiller, and Perel (1992) found positive effects, which were sustained for at least a 6-hour period, for prepubescent boys treated with pemoline.

Academic Achievement

A major issue relevant to the use of stimulant medication is whether it can improve academic achievement and learning. In contrast to anecdotal reports of parents and teachers who often insist that children show marked improvement in their school work in response to stimulants (DuPaul & Rapport, 1993; Gadow, in press; Rapport, Denney, DuPaul, & Gardner, 1994), several investigations found no improvements on standardized academic tests (for review, see R. T. Brown & Borden, 1989; R. T. Brown et al., 1997). A number of hypotheses were posited to explain this puzzling discrepancy between the observations of parents and teachers, and results from controlled trials. These hypotheses include the variability of dose response on learning, inadequate duration of psychopharmacotherapy, the use of assessment instruments that are insensitive to the effects of medication, and the possibility that the learning that takes place while children are receiving stimulant medication is state-dependent. Rapport et al. (1994) evaluated the effects of various doses of methylphenidate on the classroom behavior and academic performance of 76 children diagnosed with ADHD. Improvement in behavior, academic efficiency, and attention was associated with a linear increase in dose of medication. This is consistent with the hypothesis that dose level is an important determinant of the drug's effect on learning.

Swanson (1989) suggested that stimulants result in state-dependent learning in which information that children learn while receiving active medication is not readily recalled when the effects of the medication have dissipated. However, when state-dependent effects were identified in relation to learning, the effect is generally small and clinically insignificant (Stephens, Pelham, & Skinner, 1984).

Recent investigations continue to address the effect of stimulants on children's academic achievement and learning. In an earlier study, Vyse and Rapport (1989) examined the effect of methylphenidate on the acquisition of trained and untrained complex visual relationships in children with ADHD. Their findings suggest that methylphenidate promoted children's learning on both taught and untaught visual relations and that these improvements were similar to the changes observed in the children's attention and classroom work efficiency.

Tannock et al. (1989) examined the impact of methylphenidate on the academic and behavioral functioning of children with ADHD and found that methylphenidate results in both enhanced academic efficiency and improved behavior. Finally, Balthazor et al. (1991) found methylphenidate to affect nonspecific aspects of information processing, as measured by a classroom reading comprehension measure. They concluded that methylphenidate exerts its beneficial effects on academic processing through general, rather than specific, aspects of information processing.

The results of these studies must be interpreted cautiously because standardized assessments of academic achievement were not used. In an effort to address the limitations of previous investigations, Elia, Welsh, Gullotta, and Rapoport (1993) investigated the effects of both dextroamphetamine and methylphenidate on the performance of children with ADHD by using standardized measures of reading and arithmetic. On both medications, children attempted more reading and mathematics tasks and had an increased percentage of correct answers on the reading series. An increased percentage of correct answers for the mathematics series was associated only with dextroamphetamine.

Forness, Cantwell, Swanson, Hanna, and Youpa (1991) conducted a trial to assess the effects of methylphenidate on standardized measures of academic achievement in children diagnosed with ADHD, some of whom also had conduct disorders. Findings were generally disappointing, with the notable exception that stimulant medication enhanced reading comprehension in the group that had comorbid conduct disorder.

A significant number of children with ADHD have concomitant learning disabilities (Barkley, 1990). Moreover, attentional disturbances and problems with distractibility are frequently observed in children with learning disabilities (Douglas & Peters, 1979). This led to interest in the possibility that stimulant medications for children who have both ADHD and learning disabilities may reduce their learning disabilities. However, this hypothesis has not been demonstrated empirically.

Most studies have focused on children with ADHD who have comorbid learning disabilities. Two studies (Kupietz et al., 1988; E. Richardson, Kupietz, Winsberg, Maitinsky, & Mendell, 1988) examined the effects of methylphenidate on children diagnosed with ADHD who also had comorbid reading disorders. A double-blind trial compared three doses of methylphenidate and placebo over a 6-month period. Measures of associative learning and academic achievement scores served as dependent measures. Although there was some improvement in academic achievement, this change could not be attributed to the effects of the stimulant medication because similar improvements were noted on placebos. A similar investigation (Forness et al., 1991) found that methylphenidate had little effect on reading achievement in children with ADHD and learning disabilities. Finally, Elia et al. (1993) provided data suggesting that a diagnosis of learning disabilities was not associated with improvements in response to stimulant medication.

Most reports in the literature concur that stimulants exert little specific influence on childhood learning disabilities. The few studies that examined the impact of stimulants on basic learning disabilities were conducted primarily with children who evidenced reading disabilities. Stimulants demonstrated little or no effects on reading performances of these children (for review, see R. T. Brown et al., 1997). As R. T. Brown and associates suggest, although stimulants may have an adjunct role in the management of learning-disabled children who also have attentional disturbances, nothing can substitute for educational remediation.

The investigations that examined the effects of stimulant medication on children's academic achievement suggest that the medications exert their effects primarily on academic efficiency rather than achievement as assessed on standardized achievement tests. However, further investigation is needed to explore the mechanism by which stimulants exert their influence. In particular, whether the stimulants directly enhance learning and achievement or whether they produce changes in attitude, motivation, and/or self-regulatory strategies is an important area for future investigation.

Behavioral and Motoric Effects

Numerous studies have examined the effect of stimulant medication on childhood behaviors (E. K. Spencer et al., 1996). The literature generally reports that stimulants exert beneficial influences on rule-governed behavior and compliance to adult commands (Pelham, 1993), parent–child interactions (Barkley, Karlsson, Strzelecki, & Murphy, 1984), and physical and verbal aggression (Hinshaw, 1991). Investigators found improved maternal–child and sibling interactions (Barkley & Cunningham, 1979), as well as changes in family functioning and improved parental relationships (Schachar, Hoppe, & Schell, 1987). Much of this work made use of direct observations of children's behavior in either a classroom or a laboratory-type classroom setting (Pelham, 1993) or employed teacher and parent ratings of behavior (DuPaul & Rapport, 1993; Gadow, Nolan, Sverd, Sprafkin, & Paolicelli, 1990; Klorman, Brumaghim, Fitzpatrick, Borgstedt, & Strauss, 1994; Klorman et al., 1988). These investigations typically were meticulous in design and conducted under double-blind conditions. Generally, the results of the investigations demonstrated the efficacy of stimulants in decreasing children's disruptive behavior in the classroom, increasing time on task in completing assignments, and adhering to classroom rules (Pelham & Hoza, 1987; Pelham, Vallano, Hoza, Greiner, & Gnagy, 1992). In fact, DuPaul and Rapport (1993) provided important data to suggest that methylphenidate exerts a significant effect on classroom measures of attention and academic efficiency for children in whom ADHD was diagnosed. The effect was so strong that, as a group, the children's scores on these measures did not differ from normally developing children who were not identified as having ADHD. Similar findings were reported by Whalen et al. (1989), who found that the behaviors of children with ADHD who received stimulant medication became indistinguishable from those of their non-ADHD peers in terms of impulsivity, noncompliance, disruption, and overall hyperactivity.

In a classroom-type program at a summer camp, Pelham et al. (1992) extended the techniques of behavioral observations and controlled trials of stimulant medication. In a particularly interesting investigation, Pelham, Vodde-Hamilton, Murphy, Greenstein, and Vallano (1990) evaluated the efficacy of methylphenidate on children's attention while they played baseball. Dependent measures included behavioral observations of on-task behavior, ability to give correct answers about the status of the game, judgment during batting, batting performance, and performance on skill drills. Although stimulant medication did not improve their baseball skills, children were found to be on task twice as often while they were receiving active medication.

Overactivity has been considered a core symptom for many children with ADHD. This consideration encouraged investigators to examine the specific effects of stimulants on motoric functioning. In these studies, although the stimulants produced variable results in unstructured settings, they generally decrease activity in structured settings (R. T. Brown & Borden, 1989; Porrino, Rapoport, Behar, Ismond, & Bunney, 1983). The data on the effects of stimulants on fine-motor functioning were less clear. For example, Gittelman et al. (1983) reported significant stimulant drug effects for children identified with reading disorders who were tested with the Purdue pegboard, Raven's matrices, and Draw-a-Person test. However, Douglas et al. (1988) found few or no differences for children who were tested using a maze-tracking Etch-a-Sketch task. As R. T. Brown et al. (1997) suggested, it is likely that the effects of the stimulants on inhibitory control increase the capacity of children to delay responding, thus producing greater control over their actions and thereby improving general motoric skills.

Aggression

There is considerable interest in the capacity of stimulant medication to reduce aggressive behavior exhibited by some children. Hinshaw (1991) reviewed studies that assessed the effectiveness of stimulant medication to reduce aggressive and antisocial behaviors in children with ADHD. The review included studies that were conducted in both the laboratory in large-group natural settings. In the laboratory setting, stimulants were found to exert few significant effects. In naturalistic settings, however, stimulant medication had a large effect on aggression, according to behavioral observations in the classroom and outdoor play settings. For example, Murphy, Pelham, and Lange (1992) found that methylphenidate had a minimal effect on aggression, as assessed by a laboratory provocation task. The investigators attributed the differences in findings of laboratory versus naturalistic settings to the type of aggression sampled in each of the settings. They noted that naturalistic environments frequently elicit a mixture of both proactive and reactive peer- and adult-directed intentional and accidental aggressive acts, whereas laboratory settings typically include planned and retaliatory aggression.

Interestingly, Hinshaw, Buhrmester, and Heller (1989) found that larger doses of stimulants reduced aggressive behaviors in a laboratory setting, as compared to the dosages required to reduce aggressive behavior in naturalistic settings. Pelham, Vallano, et al. (1992) did not find any methylphenidate effect on anger or provocation in aggressive children diagnosed with ADHD in a laboratory setting. Their data further support the observations of Murphy et al. (1992), who maintained that aggression in laboratory settings was minimally affected by stimulant medication.

In classrooms, both aggressive and nonaggressive children with ADHD have a positive response to stimulant medication, as indicated by ratings of teachers (Klorman et al., 1988, 1990), parents (Barkley, McMurray, et al., 1990), and program staff at a summer camp (Hinshaw, Henker, Whalen, Erhardt, & Dunnington, 1989). Gadow et al. (1990) found that methylphenidate reduced nonphysical, physical, and verbal aggression in the classroom. There was also evidence for a contagion effect in which the presence of a less aggressive child with ADHD in a classroom resulted in decreased, nonphysical aggression by peers who were not receiving stimulant medication (Gadow, Nolan, & Sverd, 1992). Finally, some investigators (Barkley & Cunningham, 1979; Humphries et al., 1978; Whalen, et al., 1980) found that both parents and teachers responded in less controlling and negative ways to hyperactive children who received stimulant drugs than to children who received placebo.

Investigators continue to explore differences in cognitive responses to stimulant medication between aggressive and nonaggressive children with

ADHD. Matier, Halperin, Sharma, Newcorn, and Sathaye (1992) found that both aggressive and nonaggressive children exhibited similar responses to methylphenidate on measures of sustained attention, although activity decreased only in the nonaggressive group. The authors interpreted these data as suggesting that various symptom dimensions influenced by stimulants, including aggressive behaviors, are mediated by different neurotransmitters (Miczek, 1987).

A recent investigation of psychosocial, pharmacological, and combined treatments of aggressive preschoolers (Eyberg, Boggs, & Algina, 1995) provided encouraging results for an early intervention program for preschoolers with emerging conduct disorder. Pharmacological treatments included stimulant medication, and behavioral therapies consisted of a behavior management program for parents. It remains to be demonstrated whether the promising findings of this investigation, still in progress, are generalizable across settings, including school.

In summary, laboratory-based studies of young people designated as aggressive have generally suggested that aggressive behaviors are not very affected by stimulants. In contrast, investigations conducted in settings ecologically similar to classroom and play settings have provided support for the efficacy of stimulants on aggressive behaviors. The differences in findings across studies are probably due to differential assessment strategies and doses of stimulants administered in each type of setting. Replicated and extended investigations are necessary to understand the effects of stimulants on specific types of aggression.

Socialization and Peer Relations

It is the behaviors associated with ADHD that give rise to the unfavorable status and interactions these children experience with their peers (Henker & Whalen, 1989; Whalen & Henker, 1991a, in press). For example, many of these children are impulsive and immature and also disruptive with peers (Pelham & Bender, 1982). Whalen, Henker, Swanson, et al. (1987) examined the influence of methylphenidate on social behaviors in children with ADHD, ranging in age from 6 to 11 years. The study found that compared to children receiving a placebo, children who received a relatively low dose of methylphenidate exhibited less negative social behaviors when rated during unstructured, outdoor activities.

Several recent studies examined the effects of stimulant medication on the relationship between children with ADHD and their peers (Pelham, 1993) and adults (Granger et al., 1993; Pelham & Bender, 1982; Whalen & Henker, 1991a, in press). In their investigation of methylphenidate on peer relationships, Whalen et al. (1989) found that peers rated medicated hyperactive boys as more cooperative and fun to be with compared to their nonmedicated counterparts. However, despite these improved ratings in social standing, the medications did not completely normalize peer appraisals. Similarly, Buhrmester, Whalen, Henker, MacDonald, and Hinshaw (1992) found that stimulant medication muted social behaviors, decreased social engagement, and increased dysphoria in comparison to placebos. The children who received placebos were more socially negatively engaged, employed more aversive leadership techniques, and were rated less likable by their peers.

Granger et al. (1993) conducted an investigation in which adult observers rated children with ADHD who received either active stimulant medication or placebo. Children who received active medication were assessed as having passive and submissive behaviors, whereas children who received placebo were rated high on behaviors of noncompliance, aggression, and disruption. The studies also examined the malleability of adults' social impressions of children with ADHD. Undergraduate students were asked to observe two videotaped scenarios of a boy with symptoms associated with ADHD. The child was receiving either methylphenidate or placebo for the two sessions. The study found that the students combined their perceptions of the two behavior samples into a composite impression. Specifically, when the target child's behavior improved in response to methylphenidate, the ratings of the child's yet-uncontrolled behavior were quite high. These findings are particularly important as they suggest that children who exhibit symptoms of ADHD play an influential role in shaping adults' impressions of behavior, regardless of whether the children are receiving active medication.

In summary, the research is not definitive regarding the effects of stimulant mediation on social behaviors. Pelham (1993) suggested that the effective use of stimulants to increase prosocial behaviors may require the simultaneous use of behavioral psychotherapies. Greater research efforts are needed in this area, particularly studies that compare the effects of stimulants with specific psychotherapies in increasing prosocial behaviors.

Dose Effects on Cognition, Learning, and Behavior

Early studies suggested that varying doses of stimulants influenced behavior and learning differentially. For example, R. T. Brown and Sleator (1979) found that a lower dose of methylphenidate produced maximum improvement in cognition. However, the higher doses of the stimulant that were required to improve behavior had a detrimental effect on learning (Sprague & Sleator, 1977). These findings suggested that if the desired outcome is improved cognition, physicians may be overmedicating children with ADHD if they rely solely on teacher reports of children's behavior. However, results from more recent research have demonstrated that both learning and behavior reach peak effects with higher doses of stimulants (Barkley, Fischer, Newby, & Breen, 1988; Pelham & Hoza, 1987; Rapport, DuPaul, Stoner, & Jones, 1986; Solanto, 1991). Several recent studies reported that performance on cognitive tasks and classroom behavior improved rather than deteriorated as a function of increasing dose, particularly if the doses were in the low to moderate ranges (Douglas et al., 1988; Douglas, Barr, Desilets, & Sherman, 1995; Solanto & Wender, 1989). For example, Douglas et al. (1995) reported increasingly positive effects on several cognitive measures, including tests of mental flexibility, with increasing dosages ranging from 0.3 to 0.9 mg/kg of methylphenidate. Barkley et al. (1993) concluded that dose–response relationships vary among children, and thus a range of doses must be evaluated with each individual child. In general, optimal responding in cognition and behavior is likely to be reached within a "therapeutic window" of 0.3–1.0 mg/kg (M. Campbell, Overall, et al., 1989).

Summary

Of all the psychotropic medications available for children and adolescents, the stimulants are the most thoroughly studied. The primary effects of the stimulants are enhancement of attention and concentration, reduction in disruptive and impulsive behavior, and compliance with adult directives. Recent studies suggest that stimulants may also have a beneficial effect on childhood aggression and peer relationships. However, although these medications seem to enhance academic efficiency, it is unclear whether they improve actual academic achievement.

ANTIPSYCHOTICS

Generally, antipsychotic medications have been found to be superior to placebo in controlling psychotic symptoms (Pool, Bloom, Mielke, Roniger, & Gallant, 1976; Realmuto, Erickson, Yellin, Hopwood, & Greenberg, 1984). For example, Pool et al. (1976) found that haloperidol reduced the symptoms of adolescents with both acute and chronic schizophrenia, and Realmuto et. al. (1984) provided data suggesting that haloperidol reduced hallucinations and cognitive disorganization.

A more recent study found that haloperidol was superior to placebo in reducing psychotic symptoms in boys with schizophrenia (E. K. Spencer, Kafantaris, Padron-Gayol, Rosenberg, & Campbell, 1992). Children who were older, had a later onset of illness, and had higher intelligence test scores had a better response to haloperidol. Similar findings were reported by Green, Padron-Gayol, Hardesty, and Bassiri (1992).

Clozapine is a new antipsychotic for the management of childhood schizophrenia. This medication has the advantage of producing minimal adverse effects such as extrapyramidal symptoms and tardive dyskinesia (Meltzer, 1992). Mozes et al. (1994) reported on several cases in which clozapine was prescribed for children who were diagnosed with schizophrenia and who were refractory to other neuroleptic agents. Most children in the investigation experienced reduced psychotic symptoms within 2 weeks following treatment with clozapine. Similarly, Kowatch et al. (1995) reported a 42% decrease in psychotic symptoms in children and adolescents with bipolar disorder and schizophrenia who were treated with clozapine. Aggression and psychotic symptoms were the behaviors that responded to clozapine; adverse effects were documented as mild but frequent.

Schmidt, Trott, Blanz, and Nissen (1990) reported that clozapine treatment resulted in similar significant improvements in a number of children and adolescents with psychotic disorders after treatments with other antipsychotic agents failed. Gordon et al. (1994) evaluated the efficacy of clozapine and haloperidol in a double-blind trial involving 16 adolescents diagnosed with schizophrenia. They found that the psychotic symptoms abated, although a number of adverse side effects were reported with extended use. Birmaher, Baker, Kapur, Quintana, and Ganguli (1992) examined the utility of clozapine in adolescents with schizophrenia who failed to respond to other antipsychotic agents. The symptoms reduced by this agent included agitation, aggressiveness, and hallucinations. Few negative effects were reported, with the exception of sedation, which dissipated soon after the medication was withdrawn.

The antipsychotics can benefit various developmental and severe psychiatric disorders (Poling, Gadow, & Cleary, 1991b). However, for some children they may exacerbate symptoms, seriously impair adaptive behaviors, and induce disabling neurological symptoms. As a result, antipsychotic drug treatment is reserved for children with severe disorders.

Aggression

Several studies have documented the efficacy of antipsychotic agents in suppressing the aggressive behavior of individuals, including children and adolescents with mental retardation, autism, overactivity, and conduct disorders (for review, see M. Campbell, Cohen, Perry, & Small, 1989; M. Campbell & Cueva, 1995b; M. Campbell, Gonzalez, Ernsts, Silva, & Werry,, 1993; M. Campbell, Gonzalez, & Silver, 1992; Gadow & Poling, 1988; Poling et al., 1991b). Thioridazine was also demonstrated to be superior to placebo in decreasing aggression in children with mental retardation (Alexandris & Lundell, 1968). In a double-blind placebo-controlled trial, chlorpromazine was effective in reducing the overactivity of 39 school-age children (Werry, Weiss, Douglas, & Martin, 1966). Aggressiveness, excitability, and distractibility also were reduced, but to a lesser degree. In a similar investigation, chlorpromazine significantly decreased hyperactivity and aggression, according to teacher and parent ratings of behavior, while dextroamphetamines were superior to chlorpromazine in reducing physical activity (Rapoport, Abramson, Alexander, & Lott, 1971). Chlorpromazine also was demonstrated to be as effective as haloperidol or lithium in reducing symptoms associated with explosiveness (M. Campbell et al., 1993).

Werry and associates (Werry & Aman, 1975; Werry, Aman, & Lampen, 1975) provided data in two studies that haloperidol was effective in both high and low doses in reducing behavioral symptoms in boys who were aggressive and hyperactive. In an investigation of prepubescent boys who were hospitalized because they failed to respond to traditional outpatient treatment, including psychotropic medication, haloperidol was highly effective in reducing aggression, explosiveness, and overactivity (Campbell, Small, et al., 1984).

Finally, Greenhill, Solomon, Pleak, and Ambrosini (1985) conducted a controlled trial of molindone in 31 boys hospitalized due to severe aggression associated with a diagnosis of undersocialized conduct disorder. Nurses rated the boys receiving molindone as having decreased aggressive behavior. Although Greenhill et al. (1985) concluded that molindone was both effective and safe in managing symptoms associated with conduct disorder, more research is needed to confirm the efficacy and the safety of this antipsychotic for children and adolescents.

Social Withdrawal, Overactivity, and Stereotypies

The majority of controlled clinical trials of antipsychotic drugs used to manage social withdrawal, overactivity, stereotypies, and fidgetiness associated with autism have demonstrated that antipsychotic drugs are effective in reducing these behaviors (Poling et al., 1991b). In managing symptoms associated with autism, haloperidol has been found to be superior to the phenothiazines as it is less likely to cause sedation when given in therapeutic doses. In a double-blind trial, haloperidol was successful in improving coordination, affect, and exploratory behavior in children with autism (Engelhardt, Polizos, Waizer, & Hoffman, 1973; Polizos, Engelhardt, Hoffman, & Waizer, 1973). Phenothiazines and haloperidol reduced the self-injurious behaviors frequently found among children with autism (Romanczyk, 1986).

Low doses of antipsychotic agents reduce stereotypies in individuals with mental retardation. Haloperidol also facilitated discrimination learning in children diagnosed with early infantile autism (Anderson et al., 1984) and was efficacious for those children in a language-based behavior therapy program (M. Campbell, Anderson, et al., 1978). However, not all studies confirm these findings, particularly for learning on complex cognitive tasks (Anderson et al., 1989). Although haloperidol was not successful in reducing motor activity and stereotypies, it was successful in reducing other psychiatric symptoms, as rated by both parents and physicians.

Joshi, Capozzoli, and Coyle (1988) administered low-dose haloperidol to children who were hospitalized with a diagnosis of pervasive developmental disorder (a diagnosis approximately equivalent to autism in the fourth edition of the *Diagnostic and Statistical Manual of Mental Disorders* [DSM-IV; American Psychiatric Association, 1994]). Significant improvements were reported in the area of peer interactions, in addition to decreases in autistic-like behavior, aggressiveness, impulsivity, and overactivity. Adverse effects were infrequent, and cognitive performance was not affected by this antipsychotic. In fact, the majority of children were sufficiently improved to allow them to return home after hospital treatment rather than having to be admitted to a residential treatment center as was originally planned.

Stuttering

Some evidence indicates that haloperidol can suppress or diminish stuttering in some individuals (for review, see Poling et al., 1991b). To date, the mechanism underlying the effect of antipsychotics on stuttering is still unclear, although W. Fisher, Kerbeshian, and Burd (1986) suggested that haloperidol facilitates language development in children with pervasive developmental disorder.

Motor and Vocal Tics

Antipsychotic medications frequently are employed to reduce the symptoms experienced by children with Tourette's disorder. This is a debilitating neurological ailment characterized by multiple, frequently changing motor and vocal tics. Haloperidol is the drug of choice for Tourette's disorder, with about 80% of patients showing a reduction of motor and vocal tics from low doses of this neuroleptic (E. Shapiro, Shapiro, Young, & Feinberg, 1988). Pimozide is another antipsychotic that can reduce the symptoms of Tourette's disorder, and it has fewer adverse side effects than haloperidol. Shapiro and associates (A. K. Shapiro, Shapiro, & Eisenkraft,

1983; A. K. Shapiro & Shapiro, 1984) conducted a double-blind placebo-controlled trial of pimozide in both children and adults (ranging in age from 10 to 50 years) and found reduced motor and vocal tics in children with Tourette's disorder. However, adverse side effects were common and included sedation and Parkinsonian symptoms.

Cognitive Performance

A frequent and troublesome adverse side effect of antipsychotic medication in children is sedation (for review, see M. Campbell, Cohen, et al., 1989; Whitaker & Rao, 1992). Because sedation impedes learning and social relationships, there is concern about the prolonged use of antipsychotic medications in children and adolescents. This is a particular concern when antipsychotic agents are prescribed for children with comorbid learning disorders.

In their earlier observations of the adverse behavioral effects of antipsychotic medications, Fish (1970) and Rapoport et al. (1971) highlighted the sedative effects of chlorpromazine on children with psychotic symptoms. However, in a later investigation of hyperactive and aggressive children, Werry and Aman (1975) found that haloperidol facilitated performance on a number of laboratory measures, although higher doses resulted in a decrement of short-term memory. Platt, Campbell, Green, and Grega (1984) also found that for children who were hospitalized for severely aggressive behavior, higher doses of haloperidol significantly impaired cognitive performance on a simple motor task and the Porteus Mazes. Finally, Rapoport et al. (1971) found few adverse effects of low-dose chlorpromazine on intellectual functioning and distractibility, as assessed by the number of shifts of playroom activities. These findings suggest that adverse side effects of the antipsychotics on cognition and behavior are dose related, with higher doses impairing learning and school performance (M. A. Cunningham, Pillai, & Rogers, 1968; Platt et al., 1984; Werry & Aman, 1975; Werry, Aman, & Lampen, 1975).

Aman (1980) reviewed a number of studies examining the effect of chronic antipsychotic medication administration on cognitive performance of children diagnosed with mental retardation. An investigation by Breuning (1983) showed that antipsychotics depressed cognitive performance and resulted in a deterioration of learning, as demonstrated by reinforcement contingencies. However, Holden (1987) found that serious scientific misconduct flawed the study. As a result, these findings must be disregarded. Additional investigations are needed to assess the effects of antipsychotic medications on higher order cognitive processing, learning, and adaptive behavior in children with mental retardation and other developmental disabilities.

TRICYCLICS, SELECTIVE SERTONIN REUPTAKE INHIBITORS, ATYPICAL ANTIDEPRESSANTS, AND LITHIUM

The symptoms of major depressive disorder include depressed mood, appetite change (measured by a substantial increase or decrease in body weight), anhedonia, anergia (lack of energy), decreased concentration, changes in psychomotor activity or sleep patterns, and recurrent thoughts of death. Because depression only recently was recognized as a diagnostic entity applicable to children (Kaslow, R. T. Brown, & Mee, 1994), the empirical data regarding the efficacy of tricyclic medication in this population remain inconclusive (Gadow, 1992; Pliszka, 1991). Despite this, clinical use of these agents remains widespread (Puig-Antich et al., 1987). The agents can be divided into several classes, including tricyclics, selective serotonin reuptake inhibitors (SSRIs), monoamine oxidase inhibitors, and a group of atypical antidepressants.

Tricyclics

Tricyclics include amitriptyline (Elavil), nortriptyline (Pamelor), imipramine (Tofranil), desipramine (Norpramin), and clomipramine (Anafranil). Six open trials (drug trials in which either the investigators or the patients or both were aware of the medication status of the patients) of tricyclics for children with a diagnosis of depression (B. Geller, Copper, McCombs, Graham, & Wells, 1989; Hughes et al., 1990; Kashani, Shekim, & Reid, 1984; Petti & Law, 1982; Preskorn, Weller, Hughes, Weller, & Bolte, 1987; Puig-Antich et al., 1987) found that 46–100% of subjects responded favorably to treatment. However, in a series of five double-blind trials involving adolescents (B. Geller, Copper, Graham, Marsteller, & Bryant, 1989; Klein & Koplewicz, 1990; Kramer & Feiguine, 1981; Kutcher et al., 1994; Kye et al., 1996), a response rate ranging from 30% to 73% was reported.

Eleven studies investigated the effect of tricyclic drugs on depression in prepubertal children (for review, see Ambrosini, Bianchi, Rabinovich, & Elia, 1993a). All these investigations were acute treatment trials (i.e., the medication treatment duration lasted for a relatively short amount of time) lasting from about 3 to 8 weeks. Measures employed to evaluate treatment outcome included standardized rating scales such as the Children's Depression Inventory (Kovacs, 1985) or structured diagnostic interviews such as the Kiddie–Schedule for Affective Disorders and Schizophrenia (Ambrosini, Metz, Prabucki, & Lee, 1989). Approximately eight drug-trial investigations of tricyclic treatment of depression in adolescents were reviewed. Treatment periods ranged from 6 to 10 weeks. Dependent measures were similar to those employed with children and included self- and parent reports of symptoms, as well as structured diagnostic interviews that assessed the presence of a major depressive disorder.

Findings from studies of prepubertal youth and adolescents who received tricyclic drug therapy provide little support for the short-term efficacy of tricyclic antidepressants for either children or adolescents who are diagnosed with major depressive disorder (Ambrosini et al., 1993a). Ambrosini and colleagues reviewed evidence to suggest that comorbid disorders, including pyschotic symptoms and separation anxiety, predicted a less favorable response to tricyclic medication. The use of other adjunctive therapies such as hospitalization and psychotherapy did not mediate or moderate response to the tricyclic medication. The researchers suggested that duration of treatment may affect response to tricyclic medications because treatment effects may take longer to develop in depressed youth. They also posited that age of onset of depressive symptoms and current chronological age may be important predictors of response to tricyclic medication.

Sedation is a common adverse side effect, especially with amitriptyline and imipramine, and may impede a child's overall functioning at school. Several less common but nonetheless clinically significant conditions associated with the use of tricyclics include an exacerbation of mood, psychotic symptoms, and organic features, including disturbed memory, disorientation, and confusion or agitation (Preskorn & Jerkovich, 1990). These symptoms typically develop within the first 2 weeks of treatment, are associated with elevated levels of tricyclics, and affect approximately 4% of children (Preskorn, Jerkovich, Beber, & Widener, 1989).

Although some anecdotal evidence suggests that the sedating effects of tricyclics may impede school learning, there is a paucity of data on the cognitive and learning effects of tricyclics in children and adolescents. Aman (1980) reviewed the issue of tricyclics and cognitive functioning and concluded that tricyclics neither impaired nor improved the functioning on laboratory tests of short-term memory or cognitive functioning. However, Rapoport, Quinn, Bradbard, Riddle, and Brooks (1974) and Werry, Dowrick, Lampen, and Vamos (1975) suggested that low-dose imipramine may affect children similarly to stimulant medication, increasing sustained attention and inhibitory control while having little effect on intellectual functioning.

The findings support the need for continued monitoring of children and adolescents who receive tricyclic medications. More research is necessary before tricyclics can be considered a safe and appropriate treatment for children.

Selective Serotonin Reuptake Inhibitors

Since their introduction in the 1980s, the SSRIs have been widely prescribed for adults because of their documented safety and favorable side-effect profile. The SSRIs include fluoxetine (Prozac), sertraline (Zoloft), paroxetine (Paxil), and fluvoxamine (Luvox). The psychopharmacology literature supports both the efficacy and therapeutic advantage of SSRIs relative to tricyclics for treating depression in adults (Stokes, 1993).

Experience with SSRIs in children and adolescents is limited. Preliminary reports of fluoxetine (Como & Kurlan, 1991; DeVane & Sallee, 1996; D. A. Geller, Biederman, Reed, Spencer, & Wilens, 1995; Liebowitz, Hollander, Fairbanks, & Campeas, 1990; M. A. Riddle, Hardin, King, Scahill, & Woolston, 1990) suggested that it may reduce symptoms of obsessive–compulsive disorder in preadolescents and that the benefits may be sustained over time (DeVane & Sallee, 1996; D. A. Geller et al., 1995). Other controlled trials found SSRIs to be promising in reducing symptoms associated with ADHD (Barrickman, Noyes, Kuperman, Schumacher, & Verda, 1991), elective mutism (Black & Uhde, 1994; Wright, Cuccaro, Leonhardt, Kendall, & Anderson, 1995), and acquired head injuries (Jain, Birmaher, Garcia, Al-Shabbout, & Ryan, 1992).

More studies are necessary before endorsing the efficacy and safety of SSRIs for children. For example, motoric activity, anxiety, agitation, insomnia, lethargy, and decreased appetite resulting from SSRI use were reported (D. A. Geller et al., 1995; M. A. Riddle, King et al., 1990). Further, some research indicated that the SSRIs can precipitate mania and hypomania (Rosenberg, Johnson, & Sahl, 1992). One recent case study suggested the possibility of fluoxetine-induced cognitive and memory disturbances (Bangs, Petti, & Mark-David, 1994).

Atypical Antidepressants

Alternative antidepressants have received only scant attention in the pediatric psychopharmacology literature. Bupropion is an antidepressant that has limited use in children but shows some promise in attenuating attentional problems associated with either ADHD or major depressive disorder. Preliminary studies suggest bupropion may reduce the symptoms of ADHD (Barrickman et al., 1995; Simeon, Ferguson, & Fleet, 1986). Bupropion also was shown to improve memory performance in children with ADHD (Clay, Gualtieri, Evans, & Gullion, 1988), despite the adverse side effects of agitation, confusion, and irritability (Dager & Herich, 1990). Although bupropion appears to be an effective antidepressant in the management of some child psychiatric disorders, research has not yet demonstrated its safety and utility.

Lithium

Lithium has been identified in the child psychiatric literature as a potential treatment for childhood bipolar disorder (manic–depressive illness), depression, and severe impulsive aggression (Alessi, Naylor, Ghaziuddin, & Zubieta, 1994; Bukstein, 1992; G. A. Carlson, Rapport, Pataki, & Kelly, 1992; Varanka, Weller, Weller, & Fristad, 1988). Although studies of adults suggest that lithium may result in some degree of cognitive impairment (Goodwin & Jamison, 1990), there are few investigations about the effects of lithium on cognition and learning in pediatric or adolescent patients. The studies that are available suggest that lithium has little effect on cognition in children (G. A. Carlson, Rapport, Kelly, & Pataki, 1992; Platt et al., 1984). No investigations examined the behavioral and emotional effects of lithium on children who do not have a psychiatric diagnosis (for review, see M. Campbell et al., 1993). The few studies on the effects of lithium on children diagnosed with conduct disorders, affective disorders, and psychosis suggest that the medication decrease aggressiveness, anger, explosive outbursts, and mood fluctuations (M. Campbell, Cohen, & Small, 1982; M. Campbell et al., 1972; M. Campbell, Schulman, & Rapoport, 1978; Gram & Rafaelson, 1972; Platt et al., 1984). Viesselman, Yaylayan, Weller, and Weller (1993) attributed these changes to the attenuation or blunting of behavioral excesses. G. A. Campbell, Perry, and Green (1984) conducted a study comparing haloperidol and lithium on aggressive behavior in hospitalized children with conduct disorders. Lithium was found as effective as haloperidol and significantly more efficacious than placebo. Lithium also resulted in fewer adverse effects than haloperidol. There were some noncontrolled trials using lithium for aggressive children with ADHD, and although lithium did not enhance attention or concentration, its effects on aggression in these investigations were encouraging (G. A. Carlson, Rapport, Pataki, & Kelly, 1992; DeLong & Aldershof, 1987; Licamele & Goldberg, 1989). In summary, although lithium shows some promise in the management of emotional disorders in children and adolescents (M. Campbell, Kafantaris, & Cueva, 1995), more controlled trials are needed before its safety and efficacy can be endorsed.

ANTIEPILEPTIC MEDICATIONS

Antiepileptic medications, sometimes referred to as anticonvulsants, have been used for many years for the management of seizure disorders in children and adolescents. Some anecdotal evidence suggests that antiepileptic drugs may also reduce behavioral problems in children with abnormal electroencephalographic (EEG) findings in the absence of a seizure disorder (M. Campbell, Cohen, et al., 1989). However, this use of antiepileptic medications has not been systematically evaluated in controlled clinical trials. Of concern is the report in one investigation of children receiving carbamazepine for aggression. Nearly one-third of the sample developed behavioral toxicities, including mania, hypomania, impulsivity, and aggression (Pleak, Birmaher, Gavrilescu, Abichandani, & Williams, 1988). These medications are reviewed here because most children and adolescents who receive them are attending school, where the medications may affect cognition and learning.

Phenobarbital

One particularly troublesome adverse effect associated with antiepileptic medications is drowsiness. This is a relatively frequent effect of phenobarbital. In a double-blind placebo-controlled investigation, Camfield et al. (1979) also found significant disturbances in memory and diminished reading comprehension with increasing phenobarbital serum levels. Similarly, Farwell et al. (1990) reported that children who were treated with phenobarbital, in comparison to placebo, scored nearly 10 points lower on a standardized intelligence test. Intelligence was not associated with serum levels of phenobarbital, and deterioration of intellectual functioning diminished when the medication was discontinued. Based on these data, the researchers concluded that phenobarbital is associated with reduced cognitive performance.

Behavioral disturbances in children taking phenobarbital are documented extensively in the literature (Camfield et al., 1979). Brent, Crumrine, Varma, Allan, and Allman (1987) also reported a significant association between treatment with either phenobarbital or carbamazepine and the development of depression and related symptoms. It is noteworthy that when the children discontinued medication, their depression went into remission.

In summary, possible cognitive and behavioral effects of phenobarbital include decreased performance on intelligence tests and impaired memory. These cognitive processes are associated with dose; specifically, higher doses are associated with greater cognitive impairments. Other adverse side effects of phenobarbital include overactivity, emotional lability, oppositional behavior, dysthymic symptoms, and lethargy.

Phenytoin

Adverse behavioral effects of phenytoin (Dilantin) are similar to those of phenobarbital and include lethargy and emotional lability. Cognitive effects include deficits in visual–motor functioning, attentional difficulties, and deficits in problem solving. Trimble and Corbett (1980) documented a decline in cognitive functioning associated with increased phenytoin levels in a group of children with seizure disorders. However, Nolte, Wetzel, and Brugmann (1979) found no differences in cognitive performance as a function of dose. Dodrill and Temkin (1989) suggested that cognitive deficits experienced by children being treated with phenytoin were likely due to impaired motor abilities rather than to deterioration in cognitive skills, per se. Such adverse side effects are important because they may depress learning and cognition.

Thus, impairments in attention, visual–motor functioning, and problem-solving tasks, secondary to visual–motor deficits, are suggested as possible cognitive and behavioral toxicities of phenytoin. In addition, adverse behavioral effects include emotional lability and lethargy.

Carbamazepine

The literature regarding the use of carbamazepine (Tegretol) in children and adolescents has been encouraging, particularly in terms of its effects on cognition and behavior (Carpenter & Vining, 1993). Whereas some investigators attributed this improvement to improved seizure control, others suggested that the benefits may be the result of medication that is less sedating than those of other antiepileptic agents (Schain, Ward, & Guthrie, 1977).

Silverstein, Parrish, and Johnston (1982) reported some adverse behavioral effects in children treated with carbamazepine. These effects included emotional lability, overactivity, insomnia, and agitation; some children also reported mild feelings of disorientation. The effects of this medication were more pronounced in children diagnosed with mental retardation. This finding is important because these children may not have the verbal ability to describe and report symptoms. The effects were noted to be transitory, dissipating when the medication was discontinued.

Dougherty, Wright, Cox, and Walson (1987) compared children treated with carbamazepine to an age-matched, healthy control group on a series of neuropsychological test instruments. Findings were that the children treated with the medication performed more poorly in the areas of attention, concentration, and memory and were less efficient in learning novel information. Finally, in a more recent investigation, Aman, Werry, Paxton, Turbott, and Stewart (1990) found no differences as a function of dose of carbamazepine, although there was significant variability across subjects.

In summary, carbamazepine is associated with some impairments on learning and memory tasks. A less direct relationship was found between the dose of this medication and cognitive impairments than for phenobarbital or phenytoin. Similarly, reports of emotional lability, agitation, and insomnia were noted but less frequently than with the other anticonvulsant agents.

Valproate

There is a paucity of research regarding the effect of valproate (Depakote) on cognitive and behavioral functioning in pediatric populations. One study (Vining et al., 1987) reported that the effect of valproate was similar to that of phenobarbital for the management of seizures, but valproate had fewer behavioral and cognitive adverse effects. In a particularly well-controlled investigation examining low-dose versus high-dose valproate, Aman, Werry, Paxton, and Turbott (1987) found that the high-dose group had a higher frequency of motor activity and poorer performance on measures of auditory and visual integration, as well as on mazes. Again, as with other antiepileptic agents, higher doses were associated with greater cognitive toxicity. Stores, Williams, Styles, and Zaiwalla (1992) reported some decreases in attention and concentration in 63 children who were treated for epilepsy with valproate and carbamazepine. Some decreases in attention and concentration occurred with both medications. Specifically, there was a decrease in focal attention with valproate and a decrease in sustained attention with carbamazepine. However, the authors suggested that perhaps some of these cognitive decrements were a function of the seizure disorders rather than the medication.

Comparison of Antiepileptics

Some recent research compared antiepileptic medications, particularly in the areas of cognitive and behavioral toxicities. I. Berg, Butler, Ellis, and Foster (1993) compared the frequency of cognitive toxicities experienced by children receiving carbamazepine, phenytoin, and valproate. Children treated with carbamazepine demonstrated increased anxiety, irritability, sleep disturbances, and tearfulness, compared to the other two medication groups. Children treated with valproate demonstrated greater difficulties relating to separation from parents. All of these effects dissipated after 6 months of drug therapy. In a similar investigation, Mitchell, Zhou, Chavez, and Guzman (1993) compared the cognitive effects of phenobarbital with carbamazepine. Children receiving carbamazepine had committed more errors on a problem-solving task, yet they had fewer omission errors than the children who were treated with phenobarbital. Higher frequencies of impulsive errors and trends toward slower reaction times were associated with increased doses of carbamazepine.

Summary

Based on the studies reviewed, the Committee on Drugs of the American Academy of Pediatrics (1985) promulgated guidelines for monitoring potential behavioral and cognitive toxicities of antiepileptic agents. These guidelines strongly encourage pediatricians to monitor children's behavior and mood at home and school, as well as in the office setting. When adverse effects are documented, the guidelines recommend that pediatricians lower the dose of medication or consider an alternative antiepileptic medication. Further, the guidelines recommend an initial baseline assessment and ongoing monitoring of potential adverse cognitive effects by means of standardized psychometric assessment techniques and observations of behavior, including intellectual and achievement testing and behavioral ratings. In this endeavor, close collaboration between the pediatrician and the psychologist is essential.

HYPNOTICS AND SEDATIVES

Few systematic investigations have assessed the efficacy and safety of hypnotic and sedative drugs for pediatric populations. An exception to this is the corpus of studies relating to separation anxiety (school refusal) and obsessive–compulsive disorder (for review, see Gadow, 1992). Anxiolytics used for the management of anxiety disorders in children and adolescents include the benzodiazepines, antihistamines, and buspirone.

In a comprehensive review of pharmacological trials for treatment of childhood anxiety disorders, Allen, Leonard, and Swedo (1995) identified only 13 controlled trials involving anxiolytic agents. As Gadow (1992) has noted, progress pertaining to research on the management of anxiety disorders has also been hampered because of diagnostic ambiguities relating to these syndromes.

Alprazolam has been demonstrated to be moderately effective for children with overanxious and avoidant disorder (Simeon & Ferguson, 1987), as well as for pediatric cancer patients undergoing painful medical procedures (Pfefferbaum et al., 1987). Simeon and Ferguson (1987) found that cognitive functioning was enhanced with the use of alprazolam among children with overanxious and avoidant disorders. Bernstein, Garfinkel, and Borchardt (1990) compared alprazolam to imipramine in 24 children and adolescents who ranged in age from 7 to 17 years, were severely anxious, and exhibited school refusal. No differences were found between placebo and active medications, a finding attributed to design limitations and low statistical power.

In a controlled clinical trial of 12 patients who ranged in age from 8 to 16 years, Simeon and Ferguson (1987) evaluated the efficacy of alprazolam for overanxious and avoidant disorders. The follow-up period was 4 weeks. The clinicians reported significant improvements on ratings of anxiety, depression, and psychomotor agitation, and the children also rated their anxiety as improved. Parents reported a decrease in the frequency and severity of sleep disturbances. Psychometric testing of cognitive functioning also yielded significant improvements on a paired associate learning task. Adverse side effects were minimal, which was attributed to the relatively low doses of medication employed in the study. Daytime lethargy was the most frequent complaint reported.

Klein and Last (1989) conducted a clinical trial of alprazolam in children and adolescents whose separation anxiety did not respond to psychotherapy. When administered over 6 weeks, alprazolam was clinically effective: Parents and psychiatrists rated more than 80% of the subjects improved, and 65% of the subjects rated themselves as improved.

Cameron and Thyer (1985) reported a case study in which they successfully used alprazolam to treat a 10-year-old girl who suffered from night terrors. On the first night, the night terrors decreased and had not reoccurred 9 months later, long after the medication was discontinued. In an investigation designed to manage panic disorders and anticipatory and acute situational anxiety, patients who also were being treated for cancer were administered alprazolam and then rated on four scales assessing anxiety, distress, and panic (Pfefferbaum et al., 1987). The study found that adverse side effects were minimal and that improvement was statistically significant on three of the scales.

Bernstein et al. (1990) conducted a placebo-controlled study of alprazolam to treat children with school phobia. The follow-up period was 2 months, at which time almost half the children had returned to school while the remaining half showed significant improvements in anxiety and depression.

In one of the more rigorous pediatric investigations of the long-term effects of clonazepam, Graae, Milner, Rizzotto, and Klein (1994) conducted an 8-week double-blind placebo-controlled study. Diagnoses included anxiety disorder, overanxious disorder, social phobia, conduct disorder, and ADHD. No statistically significant differences were found between placebo and active medication, although the investigators noted anecdotal reports of improvements for some subjects. Adverse side effects included lethargy, irritability, and oppositional behavior, with most subjects reporting such effects.

Kutcher and MacKenzie (1988) investigated the impact of clonazepam on four adolescents with panic disorder. There were significant reductions in the frequency of panic attacks for all four patients. At a follow-up 3 to 6 months later, all the patients continued to receive the medication and had improved functioning in school and with peer relationships.

Some investigators have employed clonazepam in the treatment of obsessive–compulsive disorder. Ross and Piggot (1993) successfully treated an adolescent with obsessive–compulsive disorder for 3 months. Similarly, Leonard, Swedo, and Lenane (1993) successfully employed clonazepam in the treatment of obsessive–compulsive disorder in a young adult. Although these studies suggest the potential efficacy of clonazepam in managing obsessive–compulsive disorder, double-blind clinical trials are needed to confirm the drug's efficacy.

M. Campbell et al. (1992) reported on the use of benzodiazepines in recurrent, aggressive outbursts in mentally retarded children and delinquents and in hospitalized children diagnosed with conduct disorder. Despite some improvement in the children's behavior, the investigators cautioned against the routine use of these agents because of cognitive (e.g., memory impairments and motor incoordination) and behavioral (e.g., disinhibition, overactivity, irritability, aggressiveness, and sedation) toxicities, as well as potential for abuse, particularly in adolescents.

Antihistamines are sometimes used to reduce anxiety (R. T. Brown et al., in press) and have also been prescribed for children and adolescents to control disruptive behavior. Recent research casts doubt on their efficacy for this purpose (Vitiello, Hill, & Elia, 1991). Possible adverse side effects associated with the use of antihistamines include dizziness, oversedation, agitation, lack of coordination, abdominal pain, blurred vision, and dry mouth (R. T. Brown et al., in press).

Buspirone is an anxiolytic that may have potential to reduce anxiety experienced by children with mixed anxiety disorders (Simeon et al., 1994), school phobia (Kranzler & Liebowitz, 1988), and social phobia (Zwier & Rao, 1994). However, there were few controlled trials of this agent, and the use of buspirone remains experimental for children and adolescents with anxiety disorders (M. Campbell et al., 1993; Coffey, 1990).

Simeon (1991) evaluated the efficacy of buspirone in adolescents with various diagnoses (e.g., anxiety, depression, ADHD, conduct disorder, obsessive–compulsive disorder, and psychosis). Global clinical improvements occurred 4 months after initiation of buspirone. Improvements were noted in mood, anxiety, social interactions, sleep, aggression, concentration, and irritability. Simeon et al. (1994) also studied the effects of buspirone given over 4 weeks to treat various anxiety disorders in children and adolescents. Statistically significant treatment effects were found both 2 weeks and 1 month following medication administration. Adverse side effects of nausea, gastrointestinal disturbances, headache, and lethargy were associated with dose and were transient. Finally, Realmuto, August, and Garfinkel (1989) examined buspirone in the management of autistic youngsters for a period of 1 month. None of the children experienced adverse side effects from the medication, and two of the children demonstrated overactivity on buspirone.

D'Amato (1962) treated nine children diagnosed with school phobia who were receiving psychotherapy with chlordiazepoxide. The duration of treatment was approximately 1 month. Only one child did not attend school regularly after the second week of drug therapy. D'Amato also compared this cohort with another group of children diagnosed with school phobia who were treated with psychotherapy alone. More than 80% of the children treated only with psychotherapy remained out of school longer than 1 month, whereas the majority of children who received both chlordiazepoxide and psychotherapy returned to school The findings were interpreted to support the efficacy of chlordiazepoxide as an adjunct to psychotherapy in treating school phobia.

In another investigation of chlordiazepoxide, Petti, Fish, Shapiro, Cohen, and M. Campbell (1982) conducted a trial with nine boys ranging in age from 7 to 11 years, who had failed to respond to 3 weeks of hospitalization. The children's diagnoses included conduct disorder and schizophrenia with symptoms of anxiety, depression, impulsivity, and explosiveness. After treatment with chlordiazepoxide, two of the boys had marked improvement, four boys had some improvement, and three boys had exacerbated symptoms. Major improvements were reported in the area of verbal production, increased rapidity of thought association, and reduced depression. Petti et al. (1982) concluded that chlordiazepoxide produced the most benefit for children who were withdrawn and anxious. The child with schizophrenia had exacerbation of psychotic symptoms, and the children with severe impulsivity and aggression also had exacerbated symptoms. These data were interpreted to suggest that chlordiazepoxide may be contraindicated for children with these conditions.

Adverse side effects of the hypnotics include sedation, motor incoordination, and, according to some studies, possible impairments in learning and cognition (M. Campbell et al., 1993; Kutcher, Reiter, Gardner, & Klein, 1992). These adverse side effects are believed to be dose related. However, there has been little systematic investigation of the effects of benzodiazepines and other anxiolytic drugs in children and adolescents (Aman & Werry, 1982; Simeon et al., 1992). Research on the use of hypnotics in adults has documented impairments in the areas of memory, psychomotor speed, motor coordination, and sustained attention (M. Campbell et al., 1993). However, it has generally been suggested that long-term memory functions and untimed tasks are unaffected. The variables are affected by dose and route of administration. In memory, impairments have been demonstrated in the area of delayed recall, even when there is no evidence of sedation or other psychomotor impairments (for review, see M. Campbell et al., 1993). Finally, anterograde amnesia (blackouts) may occur following high doses of intravenously administered sedatives and hypnotics.

CONCLUSIONS

Of all the pharmacotherapies studied, the stimulants have been the most meticulously researched. Controlled trials clearly indicate that the stimulants improve attention and concentration, reduce distractibility and impulsivity, and possibly enhance peer relationships and reduce aggression. However, the short-term effects of the stimulants on academic achievement are disappointing in comparison to their efficacy in the cognitive arena. Several research questions remain to be addressed. These include the comparative efficacy of stimulant drug therapy in combination with other behavioral and educational approaches. More systematic investigation is needed to assess the effects of these medications on achievement and learning.

Antipsychotic drugs can cause cognitive impairments that may result in learning and academic difficulties. As a result, these medications must be used judiciously. However, when the antipsychotics are appropriately prescribed, they can be of considerable benefit to children and adolescents.

Because of the adverse effects associated with antiepileptic agents, it is imperative that behavior and cognitive functioning be monitored in all settings, including home and school. Ongoing systematic assessment of both behavior and learning must be the standard of care in treating children who receive this medication for seizure disorders. Because children who have seizure disorders frequently have comorbid learning and behavior disorders, it is all the more important to monitor adverse side effects, particularly in areas related to cognition and behavior. In this endeavor, the psychologist and pediatrician must work collaboratively to establish baseline assessment and monitor subsequent cognition and behavior.

Despite the excitement about the benefits of sedatives and hypnotics in treating adults with anxiety disorders, there is a paucity of data on the effects of these anxiolytic agents in pediatric populations. More information is needed about the efficacy and safety of these medications before endorsing them for clinical use in children and adolescents.

CHAPTER 4

Long-Term Cognitive and Behavioral Effects of Psychotropic Medications

♦

Although substantial information is available about the short-term effects of psychotropic medications, both in the laboratory and in classroom settings, much less information is available about the long-term effects of these medications. Most work examining the long-term effects of psychotropic medication focuses on children with ADHD and has compared stimulant-treated children with their nontreated peers or with comparison groups of normally developing children.

STIMULANTS

Results from longitudinal studies investigating the effects of stimulants with ADHD children have not been particularly encouraging (R. T. Brown et al., 1997). Researchers have examined whether children become habituated to the medication, thereby reducing the effects, and whether medicating children with ADHD during childhood predicts behavioral improvement during adolescence and psychiatric outcome during young adulthood. However, these issues are troublesome because of the difficulties associated with systematically examining the long-term effects of stimulant medication and the ethical limitations of placing children in either no-medication or placebo groups for extended periods (see R. T. Brown et al., 1997, in press; DuPaul & Barkley, 1990; Rapport & Kelly, 1991).

Longitudinal studies of children with ADHD who receive stimulants for a period of at least 5 years have generally shown that these children did not differ in any meaningful way from children who never received pharmacotherapy as a treatment for their ADHD (R. T. Brown et al., 1997). However, at the time of follow-up evaluation, the children diagnosed with ADHD were not receiving medication, which may have contributed to the lack of differences between the two groups. In a series of investigations designed to study the effects of methylphenidate on cognition and behavior, R. T. Brown, Wynne, and Medenis (1985) evaluated children when they were receiving medication and during a follow-up period when they were not receiving pharmacotherapy. There were striking differences between the findings of the two investigations. Not surprisingly, children receiving active medication performed significantly better on tasks of attention than their peers with ADHD who were not receiving active medication (R. T. Brown et al., 1985). Figure 4.1 compares results from the two studies. As shown in the figure, children who were receiving medication at follow-up continued to evidence improvement, relative to children who received placebo, no medication, or psychotherapy. The results underscore the importance of the medication status of children with ADHD at the time of follow-up.

Review of Longitudinal Follow-Up Studies

Because of the methodological and ethical problems, few investigations have studied the long-term outcomes of children treated with stimulants. Of the psychotropic medications that have been evaluated in terms of long-term efficacy, the stimulants have been the most meticulously researched. Table 4.1 presents a review of each of these.

Effects on Academic Achievement

Few differences in the academic achievement of stimulant-treated and nonmedicated children have been shown, as measured by the number of grades failed (Weiss, Kruger, Danielson, & Elman, 1975) or performance on standardized achievement tests (Blouin, Bornstein, & Trites, 1978; Charles & Schain, 1981; Hoy, Weiss, Minde, & Cohen, 1978; K. D. Riddle & Rapoport, 1976). Further, these results were independent of length of stimulant drug therapy and whether children were good or poor drug responders (Blouin et al., 1978). Overall, results suggest that stimulants do not enhance academic performance in the long term (for review, see R. T. Brown et al., 1997).

Charles and Schain (1981) examined the association between length of stimulant drug treatment and the performance of children with ADHD on tests of achievement at a 4-year follow-up. Children were assigned to different groups according to the length of stimulant treatment

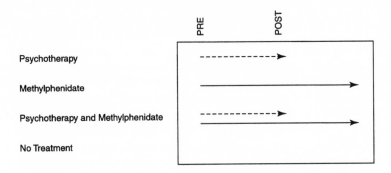

BROWN, WYNNE, and MEDENIS (1985)

BROWN, BORDEN, WYNNE, SCHLESER and CLINGERMAN (1986)

*In these two conditions methylphenidate was discontinued at post-test assessment.

FIGURE 4.1. Design of the two studies comparing methylphenidate and cognitive therapy. From Brown, Borden, Wynne, Schleser, & Clingerman (1986). Copyright 1986 by Plenum Publishing Corp. Reprinted by permission.

TABLE 4.1. Summary of Longitudinal Studies of Children Treated with Stimulants

Study	n	Type of follow-up	Type of stimulant	Duration of pharmacotherpy	Adjunctive therapy	Treatment at follow-up	Summary of findings
Mendelson et al. (1971)	83	Retrospective	Dextroamphetamine or methylphenidate	Not specified	Supportive psychotherapy	14% in clinic	ADHD symptoms diminished; 25% of the sample were reported to exhibit antisocial behaviors; 5% were found to abuse drugs; 58% failed one or more grades.
Sroufe & Stewart (1973)	83	Chart review	Methylphenidate	Not specified	Parental counseling; behavioral therapy	Treatment unclear	Children with ADHD were found to have poor self-esteem.
Weiss et al. (1975)	72	Prospective	Methylphenidate/ chlorpromazine	3–5 years	Crisis interaction/ follow-up visits at 2–4 months for medication adjustment	50%, stimulants; 11%, chlor-promazine	ADHD symptoms diminished in all groups; few differences were found between treated and nontreated children, although children with ADHD were reported to perform worse than controls in social and academic domains.

(continued)

65

TABLE 4.1. (*continued*)

Study	n	Type of follow-up	Type of stimulant	Duration of pharmacotherpy	Adjunctive therapy	Treatment at follow-up	Summary of findings
Feldman et al. (1979)	81	Retrospective	Unclear—likely stimulants	Not specified	77%, individual counseling; 37% family therapy; 62%, language/visual–peripheral training; 30%, special education	8%, stimulants; 16%, psychotherapy; 8%, special education	43% still had ADHD symptoms, 4% were in the custody of the courts, 3% were abusing drugs, 16% were found to need psychotherapy; 8% were in need of academic assistance; overall, children with ADHD were found to have poor self-esteem; some were suicidal.
Loney et al. (1981)	84	Retrospective	Methylphenidate	$M = 2\frac{1}{2}$ years	Not specified	Not specified	66% were rated by mothers as still having symptoms of ADHD; 21–29% had committed offenses against persons or involving personal property; 28% had some involvement with alcohol; 19% had used illegal drugs; 66% were 2 or more years below expected school grade levels.

Study	N	Design	Medication	Duration	Other treatment	Status	Outcome
Charles & Schain (1981)	62	Prospective	Methylphenidate	6 months–4 years	Not specified	19%, stimulants; 42%, special education; 24%, tutoring	87% of parents reported an improvement in the symptoms of ADHD in their children, while 6% reported no change, and 6% reported a worsening in the symptoms; 23% of parents and 34% of teachers reported peer problems for these children; 69% of the sample were one or more grades below their peers in reading and arithmetic; 34% repeated one or more grades.
Satterfield et al. (1981)	100	Prospective	Methylphenidate	9–35 months	41% of children, individual or group psychotherapy; 48% of parents, family psychotherapy; 29% of parents, group therapy; 57% of parents, individual psychotherapy	36%, still in treatment	Children who were treated with stimulants for longer periods were reported as having improved in all problem areas including inattention, antisocial behavior, emotional trauma, drug/alcohol use and below-grade-level academic functioning.
Satterfield et al. (1982)	110	Prospective	Stimulants (type not specified)	25 months	Brief counseling	Not specified	Symptoms of ADHD were reported as improved; 25–30% of *(continued)*

TABLE 4.1. (continued)

Study	n	Type of follow-up	Type of stimulant	Duration of pharmacotherpy	Adjunctive therapy	Treatment at follow-up	Summary of findings
							adolescents still had antisocial behavior; significant peer problems and difficulties with self-esteem also persisted; children in the study were behind an average of 2 grade levels in school.
Weiss et al. (1985)	63	Prospective	Chlorpromazine or dextroamphetamine	6 months–2 years	10%, individual or family therapy	Not receiving active medication	Medicated children with ADHD did not differ from untreated children in the area of high school academic failures, or overall grades received in high school, junior college, and and college.
Gittelman-Klein & Mannuzza (1988)	61	Prospective	Methylphenidate	6 months–5 years	None reported	Not receiving active medication	Although an adverse impact on children's growth rate was found for the active treatment phase, no group differences were reported for final height. Being off methylphenidate for two summers resulted in a positive effect on height but not on weight.

(6 months–2 years, 2–3 years, 3–4 years, and children still receiving active medication). Children who were still receiving stimulant medication did not differ in academic achievement from those children who discontinued medication. Although there were some differences among the groups at the 4-year follow-up evaluation, all the children were below grade/age expectations relative to their normally developing peers.

Only one study systematically examined the academic performance of children with ADHD as they progressed to young adulthood. In this study, Hechtman, Weiss, Perlman, and Amsel (1984) compared a group of children diagnosed with ADHD who received methylphenidate, a group of untreated children with ADHD, and a control group of normally developing children. Results suggest that the medicated children with ADHD did not differ from untreated children in terms of high school failures, grades received during high school, and junior college or college attendance.

Although further research is needed before drawing definitive conclusions, at present, there is little clear evidence that stimulant medication significantly enhances learning and achievement, as assessed on school-related measures and standardized achievement tests. Clearly, additional measures of school performance are needed, including dependent measures that assess specific abilities. Such additional assessments will enhance this body of research (Jacobvitz et al., 1990).

Peer Relationships, Aggression, and Delinquency

In the area of peer relationships, a corpus of research has examined the effects of stimulant medication on aggressive interactions with peers, sociometric ratings, peer interactions, and communication skills (Pelham & Bender, 1982). The results generally suggest that stimulant medication exerts some positive effects on the peer interactions of children diagnosed with ADHD, although Schleifer et al. (1975) have argued that stimulants result in decreased social interactions and adversely affect mood. Medicated children tend to be rated as more dysphoric than their nonmedicated counterparts (Whalen, Henker, Collins, Finck, & Dotemoto, 1979). Jacobvitz et al. (1990) attributed these negative effects to the high drug doses frequently employed in these investigations. Based on their review, Jacobvitz and colleagues recommended studies of longer duration so the long-term effects of stimulant medication on the enduring friendships and social skills of children with ADHD can be evaluated.

It has been well documented that antisocial behavior and delinquency occur more frequently in adolescence among children previously diagnosed as having ADHD (Weiss & Hechtman, 1986). Nonetheless, no differences in delinquent behaviors have been found between children with

ADHD who were treated with stimulant medication and those who were not. Among children with ADHD treated with stimulant medication for a 2-year period, relative to a comparison control group, Satterfield, Hoppe, and Schill (1982) found significantly more acts of delinquency, as evidenced by juvenile placements for the group treated with stimulants.

Critique of Studies

Longitudinal studies examining the long-term effects of stimulant medication have been criticized on a number of methodological grounds. These include the lack of sensitivity of the measures employed, especially the achievement tests (R. T. Brown & Borden, 1989; Douglas, Barr, O'Neill, & Britton, 1986; Pelham, 1986), the failure to assess compliance, individual differences of the subjects participating in these investigations, and subject attrition that resulted in biased samples.

Hechtman, Weiss, and Perlman (1984) reviewed both published and unpublished follow-up and outcome studies of adolescents who were treated for ADHD during childhood. The review focused on the effect stimulant treatment in childhood on adolescent outcome. The variables evaluated were intake criteria; compliance; adjunctive treatment in addition to medication; treatment follow-up; method of follow-up; outcome at adolescence, and type, dose, and duration of drug treatment.

The studies reviewed by Hechtman, Weiss and Perlman (1984) and Hechtman, Weiss, Perlman, and Amsel (1984) focused on children who ranged in age from 6 to 12 years, with intelligence being assessed as at least low average. SES varied considerably. Children with psychosis, seizure disorders, cerebral palsy, and hearing and visual impairments were excluded from most studies. The initial evaluations of the children participating in most studies were comprehensive and included assessments of the children and the families. Assessments yielded psychiatric, psychological, educational, neurological, and physiological data. The studies also included parents' and teachers' ratings, and some investigations incorporated psychiatrists' ratings. Dosages in the investigations reviewed ranged from 20 to 50 mg/day of methylphenidate, and medication was typically administered on an absolute dosage level rather than a mg/kg basis. The duration of treatment in the various investigations ranged from 6 months to 5 years.

Unfortunately, few of the studies reported whether or not individual children responded to the medication (Feldman, Denhoff, & Denhoff, 1979; Satterfield, Satterfield, & Cantwell, 1981; Satterfield et al., 1982), and most of the studies did not include measures of adherence. Not all studies included information about therapies or medications other than stimulant medication. Frequently, studies did not specify whether other adjunctive, nonmedication therapies were used (Charles & Schain, 1981; Loney, Kramer, & Milich, 1981). Furthermore, when alternative treatments were identified, the frequency and duration of these treatments were often not reported. Although the majority of studies did have some subjects who were still receiving stimulant medication, the presence or absence of current medication at follow-up were poorly reported (Loney et al., 1981; Satterfield et al., 1981).

Studies have employed both retrospective (Feldman et al., 1979; Loney et al., 1981; Mendelson, Johnson, & Stewart, 1971) and prospective designs (Charles & Schain, 1981; Satterfield et al., 1981, 1982; Weiss et al., 1975; Weiss, Hechtman, Milroy, & Perlman, 1985). Most of the follow-up studies included a 4- to 5-year follow-up period (Feldman et al., 1979; Loney et al., 1981; Weiss et al., 1975). Assessments included interviews with the adolescents (Loney et al., 1981; Mendelson et al., 1971; Minde, Weiss, & Mendelson, 1972; Weiss et al., 1975), other family members (Charles & Schain, 1981; Mendelson et al., 1971; Minde et al., 1972; Satterfield et al., 1981; Weiss et al., 1975), use of teacher and parent rating scales (Charles & Schain, 1981; Loney et al., 1981; Satterfield et al., 1981), and assessments of intelligence and academic achievement (Charles & Schain, 1981; Feldman et al., 1979; Weiss et al., 1975).

Most studies lacked a control group. This is a significant omission because children placed on medication may have more severe symptom presentation than their peers not treated with medication. Thus, what seems to be a discouraging picture of long-course treatment with stimulant medication may be more a reflection of the initial severity of symptoms rather than a true lack of long-term efficacy. Finally, many of the investigations reviewed reported attrition rates ranging from 30% to 50%, usually because the subjects could not be located at the time of follow-up. It is possible that subjects lost to follow-up were those who showed a better response, whereas subjects with more severe symptoms could be located for follow-up assessments. If this did occur, it would skew the results of the study in the direction of nonresponse to medication.

Antisocial behavior remained a significant problem in about 20% of the subjects, an outcome not reduced by early administration of stimulant drug therapy. However, drug and alcohol problems were not found to be significant problems, suggesting that stimulant drug treatment in childhood does not predispose adolescents to later drug or alcohol use. Poor peer relationships and low self-esteem continue to be problems for adolescents diagnosed with ADHD and treated with stimulants as children (R. T. Brown & Borden, 1989). In the academic domain, adolescents with ADHD were found to be two grade levels behind in primary academic subjects; so early treatment with stimulant medication did not seem to affect later academic achievement.

Continued rigorous evaluation of the long-term effects of stimulants remains a highly important research agenda because of the increasing use of these medications for prolonged periods, specifically through late adolescence and adulthood (R. T. Brown et al., 1997). Further, Schachar and Tannock (1993) carefully reviewed the extended treatment studies of clinical trials of stimulants with a duration of at least 3 months. They concluded that weakly designed studies with dependent measures focusing on associated symptoms rather than core symptomatology may have resulted in spurious findings, rendering the long-term efficacy of these agents less positive than they perhaps might be given better methodology.

Long-Term Follow-Up of Specific Effects

Several studies have investigated the potential long-term adverse effects of stimulant medication in specific areas. These include studies focusing on growth suppression, the cardiovascular system, tolerance and addiction, and the association of stimulant use to the onset of tic disorders.

Growth Suppression

Early reports suggested that some stimulants, including methylphenidate and dextroamphetamine, suppressed height and weight (Safer & Allen, 1973; Safer, Allen, & Barr, 1972). More recent studies reported that height and weight suppression are dose related (i.e., there tends to be suppression of height and weight with 1.0 mg/kg) and occur more frequently during the first year of stimulant drug therapy (Gittelman-Klein, Landa, Mattes, & Klein, 1988). These studies suggest that growth suppression seems to be the result of appetite suppression and is generally transitory.

Perhaps the most meticulous studies in this area were conducted by Gittelman-Klein and associates (Gittelman-Klein et al., 1988). They addressed the effects of methylphenidate and growth in children with ADHD. Specifically, they assessed the effects of methylphenidate withdrawal on the growth of children with ADHD who were assigned randomly to continue or discontinue their medication regimen over the course of two consecutive summers. After one summer, no group difference in height was found, but children taken off methylphenidate therapy weighed more. Being off medication for two summers resulted in a positive effect on height but not on weight. The investigation did not address the impact of methylphenidate on eventual adult height and weight.

In a follow-up investigation, Gittelman-Klein and Mannuzza (1988) examined the heights of young adults who were not receiving active medication but who had previously been treated with methylphenidate for ADHD. This group was compared to a nonmedicated control group who had a long history of behavior problems. No differences were found between the treated patients and controls, and both groups were at the national norm for stature.

Based on their series of investigations, Gittelman-Klein and Mannuzza (1988) concluded that methylphenidate therapy does not compromise final height, although it may compromise a child's growth during the active medication treatment phase. They explained their finding by suggesting that a compensatory growth, or growth rebound, occurred when stimulant drug therapy was discontinued. The results of these studies should be interpreted cautiously, however, because stimulants are increasingly being used for longer periods, with use extending into adolescence and young adulthood, often without significant intervals of "medication holidays." Zeiner (1995) found minor weight losses in boys with ADHD treated with stimulant medication over a nearly 2-year period. The data indicated that relatively high doses over a prolonged period might result in a failure to gain weight. Thus, although, growth suppression seems to be a transitory phenomenon with a minor, if any, influence on later height or weight, further investigation is warranted. Until the picture is more clear, practitioners should monitor a child's growth carefully, especially children who receive stimulant medication over a period of years and who also manifest low weight gain.

Cardiovascular System

In the short term, stimulants increase heart rate, respiration, and blood pressure (Barkley et al., 1993). Little information is available, however, about the potential long-term effects of these agents on the cardiovascular system. Some research suggests that these effects are transitory and dissipate with the metabolism and elimination of the active medication from the body (R. T. Brown et al., in press). In addition, although the stimulants generally have some effect on heart rate and blood pressure, these effects are usually mild (Barkley et al., 1993) and do not produce clinically significant changes in cardiovascular functioning (Zeiner, 1995). For example, although Brown and Sexson (1988, 1989) found that African American boys experienced significantly increased blood pressure following administration of methylphenidate, the boys' blood pressures remained within the normal range. Urman, Ickowicz, Fulford, and Tannock (1995) reported that methylphenidate increased the diastolic blood pressure of a group of children with ADHD and comorbid anxiety symptoms.

Of course, a major concern is that children treated with stimulants for prolonged periods may be at increased risk for cardiovascular problems during middle adulthood or later in life. Unfortunately, the follow-up studies examining the functioning of children with ADHD who were treated with stimulants for several years did not address this issue. Ethical limitations and practical considerations in research designs preclude the use of a control group over a prolonged period. This would restrict the ability to investigate such long-term effects. The long-term effects of the stimulants taken during childhood on cardiovascular functioning during later life remains an important area for future investigation.

Tolerance and Addiction

Although the adverse side effects of stimulants typically dissipate within several weeks after initiation of drug therapy, particularly with careful monitoring and dosage adjustment, no studies have yet addressed whether children develop tolerance to the drug. Studies following children who receive stimulants typically have not lasted for more than several weeks, making it difficult to assess whether tolerance would have developed in the longer term (R. T. Brown et al., 1997). If tolerance had developed, a deterioration of behavioral and cognitive performance could be expected after children cease taking the medication (Jacobvitz et al., 1990). To address this issue, studies need to evaluate children at weekly intervals during the course of several months.

Parents are often concerned about the possibility that children may become addicted to stimulant medication, particularly when it is prescribed over a long period of time. Existing studies have found no evidence that long-term treatment with stimulant medication results in addiction or serious drug dependence, when stimulant drugs were appropriately prescribed. For example, Weiss and Hechtman (1986) studied young adults who they initially evaluated as children. They concluded that children treated with stimulant medication over a prolonged period are not at greater risk for substance abuse than their normally developing peers. Other studies also found no evidence that children treated with stimulants are at greater risk for drug or alcohol abuse than children who were not medicated (Gadow, 1981; Henker, Whalen, Bugenthal, & Barker, 1981; Weiss & Hechtman, 1986). In fact, some empirical data suggest that a positive clinical response to stimulants may be associated with a lower probability of drug or alcohol abuse during early adulthood than is found in the general population (Blouin et al., 1978; Loney et al., 1981). This finding may reflect the fact that despite being in the age group considered to be at greatest risk for substance abuse, many adolescents treated with stimulants dislike taking medication and even prefer to discontinue its use prematurely (R. T. Brown, Borden, Wynne, Clingerman, & Spunt, 1987).

Although the scant research that is available suggests that the risk of addiction is fairly low, the seriousness of this issue warrants continued research. Clinicians also must bear in mind that many children with ADHD who are treated with stimulants exhibit aggressive behavior and may have comorbid conduct disorder. These children may be at a greater risk for problems associated with addiction. If adolescents have a family history that includes substance abuse, they should be carefully evaluated for the potential for addiction. If a decision is made to medicate the child, ongoing monitoring is strongly recommended.

Summary

Because many children and adolescents are treated with stimulant medication for months or years, researchers need to investigate the long-term effects of the stimulants on growth suppression, the cardiovascular system, tolerance and addiction, and tic disorders. The most well-controlled studies on the effects of these medications on height and weight generally suggest a growth rebound following cessation of stimulant medication. Nonetheless, because an association between higher doses of stimulant medication and weight loss has been demonstrated empirically, careful ongoing monitoring of height and weight should always be the standard of care. Finally, the possible effect of stimulant medication on the cardiovascular functioning of children with ADHD is an important research issue.

Investigations that examined the association between long-term stimulant medication and later substance abuse did not suggest a higher prevalence of drug or alcohol abuse during early adulthood than would be expected in the general population (Gadow, 1981; Henker et al., 1981; Weiss & Hechtman, 1986). Nonetheless, an increase in the use of stimulant medication at adolescence, coupled with the comorbidity of other psychiatric diagnoses during that age period, may place adolescents, especially those with the disruptive behavior disorders (i.e., oppositional defiant disorder and conduct disorder), at risk for problems with addiction.

ANTIPSYCHOTICS

Tardive Dyskinesia

The primary long-term adverse effect of antipsychotic medications is tardive dyskinesia, which may appear late, often months after therapy has commenced (Poling et al., 1991a). Tardive dyskinesia is characterized by rhythmic, repetitive stereotypical movements. Behaviors include sucking and smacking of the lips, shifting of the chin, thrusting of the tongue in and out of the mouth, and jerking movements of the body. Tremors of the eyelid and tongue were noted to be the earliest symptoms of tardive dyskinesia (Gardos, Perenyi, Cole, Samu, & Kallos, 1983). The symptoms range in severity from very mild to incapacitating. In severe cases, the symptoms of tardive dyskinesia can interfere with normal body functions of eating, swallowing, walking, and respiration.

Tardive dyskinesia is most prevalent among individuals who are treated with large doses of antipsychotic medication over extended periods. Prevalence rates range from 15% to 30% among individuals who are institutionalized for psychiatric disorders and severe developmental disabilities. Tardive dyskinesia is a particularly serious condition because there is no satisfactory treatment available and its effects are frequently irreversible. Although it was previously believed that antipsychotic-induced abnormal motor movements in children were qualitatively different from those symptoms in adults, recent studies have demonstrated that children display the same dyskinesias as adults (M. Campbell, Cohen, et al., 1989).

Over the past 15 years, research on tardive dyskinesia burgeoned, particularly related to children and adults with developmental disabilities, such as severe and profound mental retardation. The earliest investigation documenting tardive dyskinesia as a sequel of long-term pharmacotherapy with antipsychotic medication was conducted by Paulson, Rizvi, and Crane (1975). Since then, because of the severe nature of this adverse effect, its often irreversible nature, and frequent litigation on behalf of individuals institutionalized for developmental and psychiatric disorders, federally funded research on tardive dyskinesia has increased (Gadow, 1992; Sprague & Newell, 1987). Studies indicate that tardive dyskinesia occurs in nearly 40% of those individuals with mental retardation who are treated with antipsychotic medication. Furthermore, nearly 20% of these individuals suffer from withdrawal dyskinesia upon cessation of the medication (Gualtieri, Schroeder, Hicks, & Quade, 1986).

Review of Studies

Silva, Magee, and Friedhoff (1993), in their review of 37 pediatric cases of tardive dyskinesia, described one case of a preadolescent who was treated with haloperidol for Tourette's disorder, beginning at the age of 8. The child developed motor movements of the tongue 4 years after being adequately managed with this medication. Despite discontinuing the medication at the age of 15 years, the adolescent continued to have symptoms of tardive dyskinesia, which were associated with speech problems. This finding underscores the importance of careful monitoring of children who receive antipsychotic drug therapy, even several years into the course of their treatment.

M. Campbell, Cohen, et al. (1989) suggested several reasons for the wide variation in prevalence rates reported for tardive dyskynesia. These reasons included heavy reliance on retrospective reports, varying demographic and diagnostic factors, and differing settings where the affected individuals received treatment. In addition, the diagnostic criteria employed varied greatly. As Gadow (1992) pointed out, one of the most important advances in this area has been the development of psychometrically reliable and valid assessment scales to identify and quantify dsykinesias in individuals treated with antipsychotic medications. In fact, M. Campbell et al. (1993) recommended that children and adolescents be rated on the Abnormal Involuntary Movements Scales (M. Campbell, 1985), developed specifically for pediatric populations, before receiving any antipsychotic drugs. The authors recommended that children and adolescents be evaluated before initiating antipsychotic medication, during fixed intervals throughout the course of drug therapy, and on a weekly basis following discontinuation of the medication (M. Campbell et al., 1993).

The relationship between the dose of antipsychotic drug therapy and the incidence of tardive dyskinesia is unclear (Gadow, 1992). Two investigations failed to show a relationship between dose level of antipsychotic medication and symptoms of tardive dyskinesia (M. Campbell , Adams, Perry, Spencer, & Overall, 1988; M. A. Richardson, Haugland, & Craig, 1991). However, one review (Task Force on Late Effects of Antipsychotic Drugs, 1980) suggested that there may be an association between dose and symptoms of tardive dyskinesia. As a result, the lowest therapeutically effective dose should always be prescribed (M. Campbell et al., 1993). Finally, there is evidence that abrupt discontinuation of antipsychotic drug therapy may result in tardive dyskinesia, whereas gradual discontinuation of these medications may diminish the risk for dyskinesia (Schroeder & Gualtieri, 1985). As Gadow (1992) observed, pretreatment baseline evaluations are critical when monitoring movement disorders. This is particularly true for children with either pervasive developmental disorder or autism because it is difficult to distinguish adverse effects of antipsychotic medication from stereotypies that are characteristic of these disorders (Meiselas et al., 1989).

In a retrospective investigation of 41 children, adolescents, and young adults who received neuroleptic therapy for 1 month to 11 years, Gualtieri, Quade, Hicks, Mayo, and Schroeder (1988) found that nearly 30% of the subjects developed tardive dyskinesia either on withdrawal of the medication or after several months of treatment. Similarly, in a prospective investigation of autistic children treated with haloperidol (average follow-up was over 1 year), M. Campbell et al. (1988) reported that 30% of the children developed tardive dyskinesia. Of the children who developed tardive dyskinesia, 80% did so upon withdrawal of haloperidol (withdrawal dyskinesia), and symptoms generally appeared within 2 weeks after the medication was discontinued. The mean duration of the dyskinesias was 1 month, with a range from several days to several months. The study examined several variables for any association with development of these movement disorders: level of intellectual functioning, chronological age, gender, weight, dose of the medication, stereotypies, withdrawn behavior, and overactivity. Only gender was found to be a differential risk factor, with females demonstrating a trend toward higher risk.

Clozapine

Clozapine is a relatively new antipsychotic medication that has demonstrated potential for the treatment of psychotic behaviors in pediatric populations. A primary benefit of clozapine is that it seems to have a significantly lower incidence of tardive dyskinesia. Peacock, Solgaard, Lubin, and Gerlach (1996) compared the effects of clozapine with the traditional antipsychotic drug therapies in adults diagnosed with schizophrenia. The patients were treated for a total of 14 years (median) with the traditional antipsychotic medications and for 5 years with clozapine. Treatment with clozapine resulted in fewer cases of tardive dyskinesia.

Kowatch et al. (1995) reported on case studies of 10 children and adolescents, ranging in age from 10 to 15 years, who were managed with clozapine for bipolar disorder, schizophrenia, and other psychotic behaviors. Over a period of 6 weeks, clozapine was demonstrated to be effective in treating aggressive behavior and psychotic symptoms. Adverse side effects were mild, offering some promise for the use of clozapine in the management of aggression and psychotic behavior. Blood dyscrasia was reported to be high during the early stages of treatment (7%) but decreased to 1%, with weekly monitoring after the first 6 months (M. Campbell et al., 1993).

Although the results are encouraging, clozapine studies are preliminary, and there are, as yet, no published reports about its long-term efficacy and safety for children and adolescents. One case study documented the occurrence of seizures with the use of this agent in an adolescent with schizophrenia, so judicious use and careful monitoring are necessary (Freedman, Wirshing, Russell, Bray, & Unutzer, 1994).

Neuroleptic Malignant Syndrome

Neuroleptic malignant syndrome is another, potentially lethal, condition that may be associated with the use of antipsychotic medication. This condition is typically associated with high-potency antipsychotic agents, and the cardinal symptoms are fever, rigidity, altered mental status, and autonomic instability (Steingard, Khan, Gonzalez, & Herzog, 1992). Late effects of the syndrome may include renal failure, pulmonary and respiratory complications, and, in some cases, death (Latz & McCracken, 1992). Neuroleptic malignant syndrome typically occurs during early administration of the antipsychotic medication. However, two studies documented neuroleptic malignant syndrome in pediatric populations after long-term (6- to 9-month exposure) high-potency antipsychotic administration (Akari, Takagi, Higuchi, & Sugita, 1988; Padgett & Lipman, 1989). Thus, although the syndrome is typically associated with early high-potency antipsychotic medication administration, the results from these two investigations underscore the need for continued careful monitoring of children and adolescents for this potential deleterious effect.

Summary

The late effects of tardive dyskinesia are of greatest concern. The effects are serious, frequently disabling, and may persist long after antipsychotic medication is discontinued (M. Campbell et al., 1993). Because of the risk of tardive dyskinesia and the deleterious side effects that accompany short-term administration, few children are sustained on antipsychotic medication for long periods unless the potential danger of their symptoms far outweighs the potential adverse side effects of the antipsychotic medication. As a result, the majority of investigations that have examined the efficacy of antipsychotic medications have been acute drug trials that assessed children's cognitive functioning, learning, or behavioral response, either during the period of active drug effect or shortly after the beneficial effect of the medication dissipated. An important goal for future psychopharmacology research will be to assess the effects of long-term treatment with antipsychotic medication on children's learning and behavior.

TRICYCLICS AND SELECTIVE SEROTONIN REUPTAKE INHIBITORS

Few investigations have addressed the long-term effects of tricyclic medication in children and adolescents. The exception is the research conducted with children and adolescents treated with tricyclics for obsessive–compulsive disorder (Swedo & Leonard, 1994). The studies to date provide little support for the use of tricyclics in the treatment of depression in either children or adolescents. Also, in a 2- to 3-year follow-up investigation of depressed 6- to 12-year olds treated with tricyclics, B. Geller, Fox, and Fletcher (1993) found a high prevalence of mania in those children who received tricyclic medication. Family history of bipolar disorder was a significant predictor of the development of manic symptoms.

One study (Cook, Rowlett, Jaselskis, & Leventhal, 1992) investigated the long term effects of SSRIs on psychotic children. Although the use of SSRIs is somewhat more encouraging, particularly for obsessive–compulsive disorder in children and adolescents, more research is needed before the efficacy and safety of these medications for pediatric populations can be confirmed.

No studies have examined the long-term effects of tricyclics or SSRIs on learning and cognition. Although there is no evidence to suggest any adverse side effects in these areas over the long term, the association between depressive symptoms and cognition (Kaslow, Rehm, & Siegel, 1984) warrants future examination of the effects of these agents on learning and other cognitive processes. In short, the long-term follow-up of children treated with either tricyclic medication or SSRIs over the course of several months or years will be an important next direction for research in the area of pediatric psychopharmacology.

In a 2- to 7-year follow-up investigation of children and adolescents treated for obsessive–compulsive disorder, Leonard et al. (1993) evaluated 54 children who received tricyclic antidepressant medication. Although 81% of the patients showed some improvement compared to the baseline assessment, only 11% had no symptoms of obsessive–compulsive disorder. About one third of the variance of symptom scores at follow-up was associated with global symptoms of obsessive–compulsive disorder at the onset of the drug trial, age of onset of the disorder, lifetime history of tics, and history of parental psychopathology.

ANTIEPILEPTIC MEDICATIONS

There is insufficient empirical evidence to support the use of antiepileptic medications to manage behavioral or emotional disorders in children (M. Campbell, Cohen, et al., 1989; Evans, Clay, & Gualtieri, 1987). However, the use of these medications for children with seizure disorders is widespread, and the medication is sometimes administered for several years. This is of concern because antiepileptic medications can exert adverse cognitive and behavioral effects.

Most investigations conducted before the early 1970s that examined the neurobehavioral effects of antiepileptic medications had serious methodological limitations. These limitations included failure to control for active medication (i.e., researchers did not use placebos), measurement techniques of limited reliability and validity, and inappropriate statistical analyses (for review, see Carpenter & Vining, 1993).

Phenobarbital

One of the earliest investigations of the cognitive and behavioral effects of phenobarbital and phenytoin versus carbamazepine evaluated the effects of these medications over a 6-month period (Schain et al., 1977). The authors reported substantial improvements on tasks requiring problem solving, alertness, and sustained concentration among patients who took the antiepileptic medications. In a similar investigation involving a double-blind, placebo-controlled trial of phenobarbital and valproic acid, Vining et al. (1987) found no differences in seizure control between the two drugs, although there was evidence of neurocognitive impairments with the use of phenobarbital across a number of measures. Further, parents reported that children exhibited a higher frequency of behavioral problems when receiving phenobarbital.

For preschool children, Camfield et al. (1979) found an association between decreased memory scores and increased serum levels of phenobarbital. Further, children treated with the medication for 12 months had lower reading comprehension scores than children who were treated for only 8 months. In addition, children treated with phenobarbital had a greater frequency of nighttime sleep disturbances and more daytime irritability.

There appears to be a significant association between phenobarbital use and depressive symptoms in children (Brent et al., 1987). For example, children who became depressed after taking phenobarbital and continued to take the drug also showed symptoms at the time of follow-up, whereas children whose phenobarbital was discontinued recovered from their depressive symptoms.

These studies underscore possible adverse cognitive and behavioral effects of phenobarbital and phenytoin, including impaired memory and a general decline in intellectual functioning that was demonstrated to be dose dependent (Nolte et al., 1979; Trimble & Corbett, 1980). In addition, other adverse behavioral effects include overactivity, impaired attention and concentration, visual–motor dysfunction, lethargy, emotional lability, oppositional behavior, depression, and sleep disturbances (Brent et al., 1987).

Carbamazepine

Carbamazepine is associated with fewer adverse cognitive, motoric, and behavioral effects than phenobarbital and phenytoin, but the mechanisms underlying this are unclear. Carpenter and Vining (1993) suggested that the less sedating properties of carbamazepine may account for some of these improvements. Nonetheless, despite the improvements, studies document adverse behavioral effects, including agitation and overactivity, and some adverse cognitive effects (Silverstein et al., 1982). These adverse effects were reversed with the cessation of carbamazepine therapy. The effects were found to be most pronounced in children with mental retardation. Similarly, O'Dougherty et al. (1987) found that children who received carbamazepine for seizure disorders had greater impairments in learning and memory compared with age-matched controls. A more recent investigation (Aman et al., 1990) found few adverse cognitive effects after carbamazepine administration, although there was some within-subject variability as a function of high carbamazepine concentration levels. Thus, although fewer adverse cognitive and behavioral effects appear to be associated with long-term carbamazepine administration, studies report impairments in emotional lability and in learning and memory tasks.

Valproate

Valproate is another antiepileptic medication that has a positive effect on seizures in children (Carpenter & Vining, 1993). Anecdotal evidence suggests that valproate produces seizure control comparable to phenobarbital but with fewer adverse cognitive and behavioral effects (Vining et al., 1987). However, adverse neurocognitive and behavioral effects are associated with higher doses of valproate, particularly over a longer course of therapy (Aman et al., 1987).

Benzodiazepines

The benzodiazepines are effective in managing seizure disorders in children (Carpenter & Vining, 1993). However, long-term administration of these agents is associated with a number of adverse neurocognitive and behavioral effects, including irritability, lethargy, memory disturbances, and motor incoordination. These adverse side effects generally are associated with higher doses.

Summary

The Committee on Drugs of the American Academy of Pediatrics established guidelines for antiepileptic medication used to manage seizure disorders in children (American Academy of Pediatrics, 1985). The guidelines emphasize the need for careful monitoring of children and adolescents who receive antiepileptic medication, especially over long periods. The guidelines are particularly relevant for psychologists who practice in clinical and school settings, and ongoing observations of children's cognitive functioning, behavior, and mood in different settings (classroom, home, and playground) are recommended. Children differ in their response to antiepileptic medications, so careful observation is essential in assessing an individual child's reaction to medications.

HYPNOTICS AND SEDATIVES

The hypnotics and sedatives are a diverse collection of behaviorally active drugs, all of which have CNS depressant properties (Werry & Aman, 1993a). There is little information about long-term effects on children. Rickels and Schweizer (1995) tentatively concluded that the remissions achieved after short-term administration in adults ares frequently not sustained over time after anxiolytic drug therapy is discontinued. They further note that although many adults continue to receive sedative medication for 6 months or longer, few published empirical studies support their long-term efficacy for children and adolescents.

Chlordiazepoxide

Krakowski (1963) conducted an open clinical trial of chlordiazepoxide with 51 children and adolescents with emotional disturbances, ranging in age from 4 to 16 years. Criteria for inclusion in the study were the presence of anxiety, irritability, hostility, impulsivity, and insomnia. The subjects were kept on maintenance doses for up to 10 months. The study found that approximately one quarter of the sample had complete remission of psychiatric symptoms, and nearly one half demonstrated moderate improvement. Children with adjustment disorders were most likely to improve, whereas children with conduct disorders, "habit disturbances," and "neurotic traits" showed moderate remission of symptoms. Approximately one half of the children with mental retardation showed moderate to marked improvement. Adverse side effects were reported to be mild and included drowsiness, muscular weakness, ataxia, anxiety, and dysthymia. All of these side effects were reversed with a reduction of the dose of medication.

Kraft, Ardall, Duffy, Hart, and Pearce (1965) prescribed clordiazepoxide to 130 children and adolescents who ranged in age from 2 to 17 years. Diagnoses included primary behavior disorders, school phobia, adjustment disorder, and organic brain damage. Over a period of several months, approximately 40% of the subjects had moderate improvement, 30% had either no or insignificant improvements, and nearly 30% had exacerbation of symptoms. Children with school phobia showed the greatest improvement. Based on their results, Kraft and associates concluded that chlordiazepoxide was efficacious in decreasing anxiety, although the extent of improvement was little more than that achieved with a placebo. In terms of adverse side effects, nearly 15% of the sample had effects severe enough to warrant discontinuation of medication, and approximately 10% had milder adverse side effects that were either transient or were reversed with lowering of the dose of medication.

Summary

To date, few empirical data support the long-term use of hypnotics and sedatives in children and adolescents with anxiety disorders. Although some preliminary evidence suggests that these agents are efficacious in managing anxiety in the short term, to date that there are no long-term studies of their efficacy or potential adverse side effects.

CONCLUSIONS

Compared to the numerous well-controlled studies on the short-term effects of psychotropic medication for pediatric populations, surprisingly few investigations examined the long-term efficacy and safety of these medications for children and adolescents. Possible exceptions are investigations that examined the outcomes for children, adolescents, and young adults who received stimulant medication. Because of methodological limitations and problems with research design, these studies provide only limited information about the long-term effects of stimulant medication. In contrast to the efficacy of stimulant medication on measures of cognitive functioning in the short term, results from longitudinal follow-up studies are disappointing. Conclusions from these studies generally provide little support that long-term stimulant drug administration influences achievement. Similarly, research data provide limited support that stimulant medication improves peer relationships, aggression, and delinquency in the long run. These results are rather discouraging. However, the limitations in research design in these studies preclude definitive conclusions about the long-term effects of these agents. Multimodal trials are needed that assess the long-term effects of stimulant medication in combination with other treatments for ADHD. The National Institute of Mental Health's funding of a multicenter research program to investigate the long-term follow-up of various treatments for ADHD, including stimulant medication, will continue to be an important exemplar for future research efforts with pediatric populations (Richters et al., 1995).

Long-term follow-up studies of stimulant medications have also focused on adverse side effects of these agents, particularly effects on growth. Available data do not show that tolerance and addiction are common among children and adolescents who received stimulant medication. Research designs that test mediating and moderating factors that may place children at risk for addiction, such as family history, will form the basis of an important research agenda for the next decade.

Despite the widespread use of antipsychotic medication, particularly among institutionalized children and adolescents who suffer from developmental disabilities, few studies have assessed the long-term effects of these agents on cognition and learning. The long-term side effect of antipsychotic medications of greatest concern is tardive dyskinesia. Research provides valuable information about tardive dyskinesia and the manner in which its often irreversible effects might be prevented. The most promising approach seems to be careful assessment, both at baseline and at follow-up evaluation, paying particular attention to the administration of the lowest possible dose of antipsychotic medication. More important, because of its adverse side effects, antipsychotic medication should be used judiciously when the potential danger of the patient's target behaviors outweighs the issues of safety of these medications.

The few studies that are available generally have failed to support the efficacy of antidepressants on managing depression and related mood disorders. Although the short-term treatment of depression in adolescents with SSRIs is encouraging, the long-term efficacy and safety of these agents must be demonstrated through future investigation.

There is mounting evidence of the potential adverse cognitive and behavioral effects of antiepileptic medications. Because children need these medications to control their seizures, careful and ongoing monitoring is the standard of care. Meticulous collaboration is necessary between psychologists and pediatric health care providers to identify any cognitive or learning problems that may result from the use of these medications. Further, ongoing school consultation is imperative so that the effects of these agents on children's academic progress may be continually assessed.

With regard to hypnotics and sedatives, again, there are scant data regarding the long-term effects on children's learning and behavior. Moreover, the long-term safety of these medications is unproven. The potential for addiction is documented in studies of adults and, for this reason, judicious use of these agents with children and adolescents who may be at risk for abuse is crucial.

Finally, we are indeed struck by the fact that despite the widespread use of these pharmacological agents in school-age children, research efforts have not kept pace with prescribing practices. Additional studies employing various assessment approaches are needed to evaluate the long-term efficacy and safety of these medications across settings (e.g., at school and home). Moreover, greater collaborative efforts among psychologists, pediatricians, and child psychiatrists are needed to incorporate the expertise of each profession. In this way, careful and ongoing assessment will take place in both the clinical setting and the research laboratory.

CHAPTER 5

◆◆◆

Psychopharmacological Approaches to Treatment of Childhood and Adolescent Disorders

◆

This chapter presents a brief overview of the psychotropic medications available to treat children and adolescents with mental disorders. The discussion emphasizes beneficial and adverse treatment effects of various psychotropics through a review of some of the evidence supporting their clinical usage. The chapter does not provide the same level of detail as that found in major textbooks of child and adolescent psychopharmacology. Most of our readers are clinical or school psychologists or other professionals working in schools and clinics, and, in most instances, the medications will be prescribed by family practitioners, pediatricians, or child psychiatrists. Thus, the chapter emphasizes areas in which school personnel can play a role in the management of children receiving psychotropic medication. Such areas include discussing the potential benefits of psychotropic medication with children and parents, monitoring the effectiveness of different medication dosages, and monitoring for the presence of adverse side effects. Less emphasis is placed on the physical examination of children and laboratory investigations that must precede the use of psychotropic medication. However, physicians must complete these examinations before prescribing psychotropic medication for children or adolescents. More detailed information about these issues is available in a number of child and adolescent psychopharmacological texts (Green, 1995; Rosenberg, Holttum, & Gershon, 1994; Werry & Aman, 1993; Wiener, 1996).

A problem for physicians is the availability of a diverse range of psychotropic medications designed for adults with various mental and developmental disorders, combined with a lack of evidence of the effectiveness of these medications when used with children and adolescents. This situation increases the responsibility of physicians to ensure that psychotropic medications are used appropriately and responsibly in treating children and adolescents with mental and developmental disorders. The lack of clear guidelines for the use of psychotropic drugs with children and adolescents also increases the importance of carefully monitoring children for both the effectiveness of individual medications and the presence of adverse side effects.

As noted by Werry and Aman (1993b), a range of approaches can be employed to classify psychotropic medications. These approaches include classification based on (1) the mechanism by which the medications exert their therapeutic effect, (2) the disorders for which the medications were employed, and (3) the chemical groups or classes to which the medications belong. Each approach has advantages and disadvantages. For example, classification based on mechanism of action is useful for identifying potential new medications to manage specific disorders or predicting possible interactions between different medications. However, this system of classification is less helpful for physicians who primarily wish to know the range of medications available to treat particular disorders; for them, classification based on therapeutic usage typically is more useful.

At present, classification based on therapeutic usage generally groups psychotropic medications according to their effectiveness in managing adult psychiatric disorders. However, the medication groups derived on this basis and the summary terms used to describe them are often less appropriate for grouping psychotropic medications employed to treat child and adolescent psychiatric and developmental disorders. For example, the term *antidepressants* often is used to describe a group of medications that are used to treat depressive disorders experienced by adults. At present, however, there is little evidence that the medications in this group are effective for treating depressive disorders experienced by children and adolescents. As a result, in the context of child and adolescent psychopharmacology, it is difficult to justify using the term *antidepressants* to describe the group. However, terms such as *antidepressants* or *anxiolytics* are so pervasive in the psychopharmacology literature that it is also difficult to justify the use of an alternative classification in this book.

Waters (1990) noted several advantages of basing reviews of child and adolescent psychopharmacology on medication classes rather than on the mental disorders the medications treat. First, better quality information is available about the nature of the medications and their clinical effects than about their effectiveness in managing specific disorders. The clinical effects also tend to be the same, regardless of the disorder being treated. Second, there is often a discrepancy between evidence of the effectiveness of different medications and their actual use to treat childhood mental disorders in the community. For example, despite limited evidence of the effectiveness of tricyclic antidepressant medication to treat childhood depression, physicians appear to use the tricyclics widely for this purpose. Finally, there is great variation in the quality of evidence supporting the effectiveness of different medications for specific disorders. Commonly, evidence is based on anecdotal data, including case reports or open trials, with only a small number of double-blind placebo-controlled trials available to guide prescribers. This paucity of solid evidence of effectiveness makes it difficult to convey accurately the efficacy of psychotropic drugs when reviews are based on treatment groups rather than on medication classes.

Psychotropic medications tend to be employed in one of two ways with children and adolescents. One approach employs psychotropic medications primarily to reduce target symptoms. An example is the use of psychotropic medications to reduce aggressive behavior or anxiety symptoms, which are common features of several childhood psychiatric disorders. The other approach employs psychotropic medications to treat childhood mental disorders or syndromes, anticipating that the medication will have a beneficial effect across the broad range of symptoms comprising a specific psychiatric disorder. An example is the use of phenothiazine medication to treat childhood schizophrenia, with the expectation that the medication will reduce symptomatology in a range of areas. It is important for psychologists to know which prescription approach is being employed when they discuss the use of psychotropic drugs with children or parents.

DEVELOPMENTAL ISSUES RELEVANT TO PRESCRIBING PSYCHOTROPIC MEDICATIONS FOR PEDIATRIC POPULATIONS

Children are both qualitatively and quantitatively different from adults. Thus, a number of issues different from those that apply to adults must be considered when prescribing and monitoring medication for children.

Physiological Factors

Physiologically, children are not simply small adults. For example, the rate at which medications are absorbed, distributed in the body, and metabolized by children can differ dramatically from those processes in adults

(Paxton & Dragunow, 1993). As a result, clinicians must take great care when they decide on the initial medication dosages and any dosage changes during the course of treatment. For these reasons, parents must always consult the physician who is prescribing a child's medication before altering dosages. Similarly, to avoid medication interactions that may adversely affect children, parents should always consult a child's physician before employing new medications for children.

Psychological Factors

Young children are less able than adults to describe with accuracy the changes in their physical or psychological functioning arising from the use of psychotropic medications, the nature of adverse side effects associated with psychotropic medications, and the time course of these changes or adverse side effects. These are important issues, particularly when psychotropic medications are being used to reduce feelings or symptoms of depression or anxiety. There is considerable evidence that the level of agreement between child, parent, and teacher reports of children's internalizing symptoms is relatively poor (Achenbach, McConaughy, & Howell, 1987). Thus, it is essential that information be obtained from all three informants (i.e., children, parents, and teachers) to assess the beneficial and adverse effects of psychotropic medication used to treat childhood anxiety or depression.

Adherence to Medication Regimens

Compliance with recommended dosage schedules is a major factor which can influence the effectiveness of drug treatment. Many issues make prescribing medication for children more complicated than prescribing for adults. For example, children are almost always brought to physicians because parents or school staff are concerned that a child has problems that must be treated. Children do not arrange their own appointments to see a physician. As a result, unless they fully understand the benefits to their health and functioning, children may be reluctant to use psychotropic medication.

In most cases, parents rather than children take responsibility for the administration of children's medication. As a result, parental attitudes may also influence children's use of medication. Some parents may be reluctant to use medication for their children if school staff initiated the referral and the children's behavior is not causing problems at home. Children who receive medication while attending school may also believe that they are being labeled or singled out by school staff. As a result, they may be reluctant to comply with treatment. Chapter 7 presents a more extended discussion on adherence to pharmacological treatments.

School staff can play an important role in assisting children and parents in understanding the nature of children's medication and encouraging compliance with recommended dosage schedules. Nurcombe and Partlett (1994) have provided a useful summary of several issues that should be discussed with parents and children. These include (1) the nature of the condition that requires treatment, (2) the purpose of the proposed treatment and the probability that it will succeed, (3) the risks and consequences of the proposed pharmacological treatment, (4) alternatives to the proposed treatment and their attendant risks and consequences, and (5) prognosis with and without the proposed treatment.

It is essential that school personnel liaise closely with the prescribing physicians to ensure that advice about medication is consistent. This liaison is particularly important if school personnel are involved in other aspects of children's treatment programs, such as remedial education or behavior modification programs. Children and parents may easily become confused if they receive conflicting information from teachers, psychologists, and physicians. Such conflicts can undermine the confidence of children and parents in treatment programs and contribute to poor adherence. To overcome these problems, regular contact between the children's physicians and school personnel is essential.

Coordination with Other Treatment Programs

In most instances, psychotropic medications are only one element of children's treatment programs. Typically, psychotropics are employed to reduce children's symptomatology with the expectation that this reduction will facilitate the effectiveness of other psychological, social, or educational interventions. School staff often play a key role in the delivery of these interventions. As a result, they are well placed to coordinate treatment with psychotropic medications and other therapies focusing on the psychological, social, or educational problems experienced by children.

Summary

A number of special issues are associated with prescribing psychotropic medication to pediatric populations. These issues include developmental considerations that are unique to children and adolescents, compliance with psychopharmacological treatment regimens, and the coordination of other treatment programs that are frequently employed along with drug treatment.

USE OF PSYCHOTROPICS

Stimulants

The report published by Bradley (1937), which described the use of stimulant medication to treat behaviorally disordered children, represents one of the first attempts to evaluate the effectiveness of a psychotropic medication for a childhood psychiatric disorder. Since Bradley's report, a vast literature has emerged describing the use of stimulant medication with children. There is also increasing interest in the potential use of these medications with adolescents and adults, although less information is available about the effectiveness of stimulant medications with these age groups (Klormanet al., 1990).

This group of stimulants is composed primarily of three medications: methylphenidate (Ritalin), dextroamphetamine (Dexedrine), and pemoline (Cylert). Currently, these are the most commonly prescribed medications for childhood psychiatric disorders. For example, estimates indicate that nearly 2% of the school-age population in the United States receive stimulant medication for ADHD, and the rate of prescriptions doubled every 4 to 7 years during the 1980s (Barkley, 1990; Safer & Krager, 1988).

Pharmacology and Pharmacokinetics

Table 5.1 presents information about the dose, actions, and half-life of the three stimulants used for children. Researchers believe that the stimulants work by enhancing catecholamine activity in CNS. Amphetamines appear to stimulate the release of biogenic amines from their storage sites in nerve terminals, thus increasing their availability in the synaptic cleft (Hardman, Limbird, Molinoff, Ruddon, & Gillman, 1996). Although the mechanisms of action of methylphenidate and pemoline are less well understood, it seems likely that they have similar effects at the synapses (Barkley et al., 1993). However, a broad neurophysiological understanding of the method by which the medications affect children's cognition and behavior has yet to be achieved (Pliszka, McCracken, & Maas, 1996).

Stimulants are almost always administered orally. They are quickly absorbed and then rapidly eliminated from the body. Methylphenidate reaches a peak plasma level in children within 1.5–2.5 hours, and dextroamphetamine reaches a peak plasma level within 2–3 hours after ingestion. Pemoline reaches a peak plasma concentration within 2–4 hours of ingestion, but appears to have a somewhat longer plasma half-life and remains effective within the body for a longer period of time than the other

TABLE 5.1. Commonly Used Stimulants in Children and Adolescents

	Dextroamphetamine (Dexedrine)	Methylphenidate (Ritalin)	Pemoline (Cylert)
	Overactivity, impulsivity, and inattention indications		
How supplied (mg)	5; SP 5, 10, 15	5, 10, 20; SR 20	18.75, 37.5, 75
Single-dose range (mg/kg)	0.15–0.5	0.3–0.7	0.5–2.5
Daily dose range			
mg/kg/day	0.3–1.25	0.6–2.0	0.5–3.0
mg/day	5–40	10–60	18.75–112.5
Initial single dose	2.5 mg, two to three times/day	5 mg, two to three times/day	18.75 mg each morning
Peak plasma level	2–3 hours	1.5–2.5 hours	2–4 hours
Plasma half-life	4–6 hours	2–3 hours	7–8 hours (children)
Peak clinical effect	1–2 hours	1–3 hours	If prescribed as indicated, several weeks after treatment begins; therapeutic effect is generally sustained over several hours
Onset of behavioral effect	30–60 minutes	30–60 minutes	Variable
Duration of behavioral effect	4–6 hours	3–5 hours	6–8 hours
Common adverse reactions	Difficulty in falling asleep and mild elevation of pulse and blood pressure		
Less frequent adverse reactions	Decreased appetite (temporary), crying and dysphoria, growth retardation (height and weight, mild), drowsiness, anxiety, and irritability		
Serious but unusual adverse reactions	Psychotic thoughts, lowering seizure threshold, worsening of tic disorder or dyskinesia, potential for medication abuse, and hypertension		As with Dexedrine and Ritalin, plus hepatocellular injury, elevated serum glutamic pyruvic transaminase

Note. SP, spansule; SR, sustained release.

two stimulant medications. As a result, pemoline only has to be administered once a day. The other two stimulants are generally administered twice daily; however, sustained-release versions with more prolonged action than the regular versions are available. The slow-acting form of methylphenidate is known as Ritalin-SR and the version for dextroamphetamine is Dexedrine Spansule. (See Table 5.1.)

Clinical Effects

A vast literature describes the clinical effects of the stimulant medications (for review, see Barkley, 1990; Gadow, 1992). This section summarizes the most relevant effects for the management of children with problems at school where the key benefits of stimulant medications are their ability to reduce impulsivity, improve sustained attention to assigned tasks, and reduce restless behavior (Rapport et al., 1994). In practice, these effects mean that the medications can improve the on-task behavior of children with ADHD and reduce classroom disruptiveness (Pelham, 1993).

The stimulants produce positive effects on sustained and persistent efforts to accomplish assigned tasks. They also reduce task-irrelevant restlessness and motor activity (Barkley, 1977; Barkley et al., 1993; Jacobvitz et al., 1990). There also is compelling evidence that the stimulants significantly reduce hyperactivity in children and adolescents with ADHD (Barkley, 1990). Further, stimulants increase children's compliance with parental commands and improve children's interpersonal relations with peers (Pelham, 1993; Rosenberg et al., 1994). Stimulants also reduce the intensity and improve the quality of social interaction between children with ADHD and their parents and teachers (Barkley et al., 1993). Finally, children receiving stimulants exhibit reduced aggression in school settings (Gadow et al., 1990; Hinshaw, 1991).

It is difficult to reach definitive conclusions about the cognitive effects of the stimulant medications. Gadow (1992) noted that there are numerous measures of cognitive performance and that simple modifications to the same cognitive task may generate quite different patterns of medication effects. Thus, despite compelling evidence that stimulants enhance sustained attention and reduce distractibility and hyperactivity in children, their effects on the cognitive functioning of children is unclear. Earlier studies suggested that the stimulants did not improve children's academic performance; however, increasing evidence suggests that, at least in the short term, stimulants can improve academic functioning (C. L. Carlson, Pelham, Milich, & Dixon, 1992; Douglas et al., 1988). What remains less clear is whether stimulant medication improves children's academic performance over the long term (Hinshaw, 1991; Jacobvitz et al., 1990). High dosages of stimulants may reduce children's cognitive ability, a side effect that may be apparent first to school staff. Chapters 3 and 4 present a more detailed discussion of the short- and long-term cognitive and behavioral effects of stimulant medication.

Adverse Side Effects

School staff can play a key role in monitoring the effects of stimulant medication because they have the opportunity to observe children over long periods of time in both structured classroom settings and less structured playground activities. Moreover, the presence of large numbers of children of the same age and sex enables school staff to compare the behavior of children who are receiving medication with the behavior of their peers who are not being treated with pharmacotherapy. Although a number of adverse side effects are described with stimulant medication, most are not severe and generally cease when medication is discontinued or the dosage is reduced (see Table 5.2).

Barkley, McMurray,et al. (1990) conducted a trial of stimulant medication in which a substantial proportion of the children who received placebo were reported to have side effects. They concluded that, for some children, symptoms attributed to side effects may in fact be part of the child's disorder or arise from the process of using medication (see Table 5.3).

Specific adverse side effects of stimulants include insomnia, anorexia or weight loss, abdominal pain, motor tics or nervous movements, and

TABLE 5.2. Untoward Effects of Stimulant Medication

Frequent	Uncommon
Decreased appetite	Cognitive impairment
Gastrointestinal pain	Dizziness, lethargy, fatigue
Increased heart rate	Insomnia
(clinically insignificant)	Growth retardation
Irritability	Hyperacusis
Paradoxical worsening of behavior	Impaired liver functioning (pemoline only)
	Increased blood pressure
	Increased heart rate (clinically significant)
	Major depressive episodes
	Nausea, constipation
	Rash/hives
	Psychosis
	Sadness/isolation
	Tic disorders (i.e., Tourette's syndrome)

Note. Adapted from Rosenberg et al. (1994). Copyright 1994 by Taylor & Francis. Adapted by permission.

TABLE 5.3. Percentage of 82 Subjects (Rated by Parents) Displaying Side Effects of Methylphenidate Given at Two Doses

	Percentage[a]					
			Dose of active medication			
	Placebo		Low[b]		Medium[c]	
Side effects	Total	Severe	Total	Severe	Total	Severe
Decreased appetite	15	1	52	7	56	13
Insomnia	40	7	62	18	68	18
Stomachaches	18	0	39	1	35	6
Headaches	11	0	26	1	21	4
Prone to crying	49	10	59	16	54	10
Tics and nervous movements	18	4	18	7	28	5
Dizziness	4	0	10	0	7	1
Drowsiness	18	1	23	2	20	1
Nail biting	22	7	26	4	29	9
Talks less	16	1	20	1	22	2
Anxiousness	58	12	58	9	52	7
Disinterested in others	18	0	18	1	15	2
Euphoria	41	9	34	4	43	7
Irritable	72	18	65	15	66	13
Nightmares	20	0	20	0	21	3
Sadness	43	5	48	6	41	8
Staring	40	2	38	4	38	1

Note. Adapted from Barkley, McMurray, et al. (1990). Copyright 1990. Reproduced by permission of *Pediatrics,* Vol. 86, No. 2, pp. 184–192, August 1990.

[a]Percentage total refers to the number of subjects rated a 1 or higher on the scale of severity (1–9), whereas percentage severe refers to the number of subjects whose severity rating was 7 or higher (7–9).

[b]0.3 mg/kg.

[c]0.5 mg/kg.

cognitive toxicities. Insomnia is one of the most common adverse side effects of the stimulants. Barkley, McMurray, et al. (1990) reported that more than 50% of children with ADHD who were receiving methylphenidate developed insomnia. Anorexia and weight loss are other commonly reported adverse side effects. Of concern is the possibility that the long-term use of stimulants may retard the growth of children. On balance, it appears that some growth reduction may occur (Jacobvitz et al., 1990). What is less clear is whether later growth fully compensates for this initial delay. In light of this uncertainty, it is important to monitor children's height and weight while they are receiving stimulant medication. In addition, every effort should be made to minimize the total amount of medication children receive. This result can be achieved by refraining from administering medication to children when their behavior does not require it, for example, on weekends or school holidays. Careful consultation with parents is necessary when minimizing medication this way. Chapter 4 presents additional information pertaining to the long-term effects of the stimulants on height and weight.

Although abdominal pain is reported as a common adverse side effect, approximately 18% of children who were receiving a placebo in the study reported by Barkley, McMurray, et al. (1990) also described this effect. The onset of motor tics or involuntary motor movements is an uncommon adverse side effect. However, when it does occur, medication should be discontinued. School personnel are in an excellent position to observe this adverse side effect.

Tics

One body of literature has suggested an association between tics and the use of stimulant medication (Caine, Ludlow, Polinsky, & Ebert, 1984; Feinberg & Carroll, 1979; Meyerhoff & Snyder, 1973). For this reason, children with Tourette's disorder or children with a family history of tics or Tourette's disorder are cautioned against using stimulant medication (Barkley, McMurray, et al., 1990; D. J. Cohen & Leckman, 1989; Golden, 1985). Other studies indicated that short-term stimulant drug therapy does not result in increased severity of tic symptoms (Castellanos & Rapoport, 1992; Gadow et al., 1992; Sverd, Gadow, & Paolicelli, 1989). Although these recent investigations offer some encouragement for the safe use of stimulant medication without undue concern about tics, based on the review of investigations that yielded mixed results (M. A. Riddle et al., 1995; Sverd, Gadow, Nolan, Sprafkin, & Ezor, 1992; Voeller, Marcus, & Lewis, 1993), ongoing monitoring should be the standard of care. Until such studies examining the long-term effects of stimulants on the production or exacerbation of tics are forthcoming and definitive, caution should be the rule rather than the exception. Because children and adolescents may receive stimulant medication for months or years, the practitioner must carefully evaluate for the presence of tics.

Several other adverse side effects have been described, including tearfulness, headaches, and irritability. It is unclear whether irritability is a direct effect of the medication, a "rebound" phenomenon that may occur when medication ceases to be effective, or simply a return to baseline behavior that was present before introduction of the medication. Finally, pemoline may be associated with skin rashes and with a chemical hepatitis (a disease of the liver). Recent communications disclosed 10 reports in the United States of acute liver failure in children, with additional reports of liver failure in adults and in children from foreign countries (Abbott Pharmaceuticals, 1996). This figure represents 4 to 17 times the rate expected in the general population. Of the 13 cases of liver failure that were reported as of 1996, 11 resulted in death or liver transplantation within 4 weeks of the onset of signs and symptoms of liver failure. Based on discussions with the Food and Drug Administration (FDA), it is recommended that pemoline should not ordinarily be considered a first-line drug therapy for children diagnosed with ADHD (Abbott Pharmaceuticals, 1996).

Contraindications and Medication Interactions

Traditionally, a history of tics, Tourette's disorder, or psychosis contraindicated the use of stimulants (Barkley et al., 1993). Recently, however, Gadow, Sverd, Sprafkin, Nolan, and Ezor (1995) suggested that methylphenidate is a safe medication for the treatment of ADHD for the majority of children with a history of tics. Nonetheless, caution is necessary when stimulants are used in families with a history of medication abuse or in children who have experienced problems with their growth. Finally, children with a history of liver disorders should not be treated with pemoline because of the risk of liver dysfunction.

Dosage and Administration

In the past, it was suggested that there are no good predictors of stimulant medication response (Jacobvitz et al., 1990). However, Buitelaar, Van der Gaag, Swaab-Barneveld, and Kuiper (1995) recently suggested that a combination of high mental abilities, considerable inattentiveness, younger age, low severity of disorder, and low rates of anxiety predicted a better response to methylphenidate. The presence of internalizing symptoms (e.g., depression and anxiety) may predict a poorer response to methylphenidate (DuPaul, Barkley, & McMurray, 1994).

Few factors predict a good response to a specific stimulant medication and few guidelines identify specific stimulants that should initially be employed to treat an individual child. However, Barkley et al. (1993) recommended that methylphenidate should generally be the initial stimulant employed to treat children because of its proven efficacy across a wide age range and the corpus of data about its beneficial and adverse side effects. However, the failure of a child to respond to one stimulant medication does not necessarily predict a poor response to others. As a result, if a child does not respond to methylphenidate, it is quite appropriate to undertake a subsequent trial of dextroamphetamine or pemoline. In general, because it has potentially more severe adverse side effects, pemoline should not be the first stimulant employed to treat a child with ADHD.

The rapid absorption and elimination of dextroamphetamine and methylphenidate have several treatment implications for school staff. First, it is important to ensure that these medications are administered at a time that ensures their peak effectiveness when the target symptoms are most problematic (Pelham, 1993). For example, if a child's behavior is most problematic in the morning, medication should be administered at the beginning of the day. Unfortunately, parents may then receive little respite from their children's problematic behavior at the end of the day because of the drugs' short period of action.

Poor compliance with prescribed medication regimes is a common problem and, in part, may explain the variable effects of stimulant medication. As a result, it is essential that school staff achieve a close working relationship with parents to ensure that children receive the prescribed medication dosages at the correct time of the day. The need to adjust medication dosages also requires close collaboration between school staff—who are in the best position to observe the effects of different dosages on children's behavior—and physicians who are prescribing the stimulant medication. The rapid elimination of stimulant medication also makes it likely that many children will require a dose at lunch time. It is important that this process be handled sensitively to ensure that children are not embarrassed by the procedure or teased by their peers. If this occurs, children may refuse to take their medication.

It is difficult for a physician to judge the effects of different medication dosages when the child's problems occur primarily at school. Children typically are brought to a doctor's appointment by their parents, who rarely observe children's behavior at school. As a result, parents' reports are limited to information they receive from their child's teachers. Appointments with physicians are typically short and take place in office settings that provide little opportunity to observe the child's behavior. To overcome these problems, it is essential that school staff provide regular reports to physicians about a child's school-based behavior problems.

The effect of stimulants may vary greatly across individual children and within children; the same dose of a medication may have different effects on various symptoms (Barkley et al., 1993; Rapport et al., 1994). As a result, it is important to clarify which symptoms are being targeted, to vary the dosage of medication across an appropriate range of levels to achieve maximum effectiveness, and to monitor carefully the effect of the medication on the target symptoms. Because stimulant medication has a short half-life, trials to test the effectiveness of these drugs can include daily changes of both medication dosage and placebo (Pelham, 1993). Pelham suggested that a controlled trial of medication should include a rotating regimen of medication and placebo over several weeks to identify the most effective dose of medication. Several useful guides are available to help physicians and school staff in this area (Barkley et al., 1993; Gadow & Nolan, 1993; Pelham, 1993).

Summary

The stimulants represent the most widely used class of psychotropic medications for children and adolescents. They are short-acting agents that are administered orally, and their beneficial effects include enhancing sustained attention and decreasing restless behavior, distractibility, overactivity, and impulsivity. Their side effect profiles are generally short term and primarily involve insomnia, anorexia or weight loss, and abdominal pain. Because of their short half-life, the efficacy of the stimulants may easily be evaluated, particularly within classroom situations.

Although the stimulants have been studied extensively, many unanswered questions remain. One particular issue is the effectiveness of multimodal treatment strategies that combine psychosocial and pharmacological approaches. The relative success of medication compared to the combination of medication and behavioral therapy remains to be substantiated empirically. The current six-site multimodal treatment study of ADHD sponsored by the National Institute of Mental Health and the U.S. Department of Education is expected to provide answers to this question some time in 1998. Questions also remain about the emanative effects of stimulant drug treatment and whether changes in self-perception occur if improvement is attributed to medication (Whalen & Henker, in press). Finally, Whalen and Henker urge further research on treatment acceptability, adherence, and satisfaction with stimulant use. This is an important research direction for this area.

Antipsychotics

The antipsychotic drugs are a large group of psychoactive medications used to treat severe psychiatric disorders experienced by adults, including schizophrenia and mania. The medications may be classified into groups on the basis of either their chemical structure or their potency for neurotransmitters at specific receptor sites. Table 5.4 shows a common grouping of these medications.

The first antipsychotic medications were identified in the 1950s. These were the phenothiazines, of which chlorpromazine was the prototype. A new high-potency group of medications was later identified in the early 1960s, when it was recognized that the extent to which drugs could achieve a blockade of dopamine receptors was a key element in determining their effectiveness as antipsychotic medications. This group of medications, which includes haloperidol, caused less sedation and fewer adverse cardiovascular effects but was more commonly associated with adverse neurological effects. More recently, new medications with fewer adverse neurological effects have become available, including such drugs as cloza-

TABLE 5.4. Grouping of Antipsychotic
Medications

Compound	Trade name
Phenothiazines	
Chlorpromazine	Thorazine
Thioridazine	Mellaril
Mesoridazine	Serentil
Trifluoperazine	Stelazine
Fluphenazine	Prolixin
Perphenazine	Trilafon
Prochloperazine	Compazine
Thioxanthenes	
Chlorprothixene	Taractan
Thiothixene	Navane
Indolic compounds	
Molindone	Moban
Diphenylbutylipiperdines	
Pimozide	Orap
Butyrophenones	
Haloperidol	Haldol
Droperidol	Inapsine
Dibenzoxapines	
Loxapine	Loxitane
Clozapine	Clozaril

Note. Adapted from Rosenberg et al. (1994). Copyright
1994 by Taylor & Francis. Adapted by permission.

pine and risperidone. Clozapine has a different mechanism of action than
the standard antipsychotics and is proving to be useful for adults experiencing treatment-resistant schizophrenia. To date, there are only limited
reports of its effectiveness when used with children and adolescents
(Birmaher et al., 1992; McClellan & Werry, 1994).

Poling, Gadow, and Cleary (1991b) estimated that hundreds of millions of children, adolescents, and adults have been treated with these
medications since the agents were first marketed in the 1950s. They suggested that the availability of antipsychotic drugs has had an extraordi-
nary benefit for individuals with mental illness. Among adults, the drugs
have changed the environment of psychiatric hospitals and residential institutions for the retarded by decreasing physical assaults on staff, decreasing destruction of property, and reducing the amount of time that patients
spend in restraints and seclusion. Many adult patients are able to leave
psychiatric hospitals, return home, and receive outpatient treatment at
community mental health agencies.

It is important for school staff to know whether children are being treated with antipsychotic medications because the drugs can have a significant effect on children's school work, and children and adolescents may experience severe adverse side effects. For example, the sedative effect of low-potency medications can interfere with children's work at school, and adolescents receiving high-potency medications may experience severe adverse neurological effects. School staff can play a vital role in monitoring for these potentially debilitating problems. Such monitoring can be a major challenge for school staff responsible for children with chronic psychiatric disorders who may have to be monitored for several years.

Pharmacology and Pharmacokinetics

Abnormalities of neurotransmitter systems play an important role in the etiology of major psychiatric disorders, and the effectiveness of antipsychotic medications appears to reflect their ability to overcome these abnormalities (Hardman et al., 1996). There is little information about the absorption and metabolism of antipsychotic drugs in children and adolescents. However, studies of adults suggest considerable variation in the rate of absorption and elimination of these medications, particularly when they are administered orally. In addition, the medications may continue to have pharmacological effects several days after they are discontinued. Because of the lack of information about the effect of antipsychotic drugs on the younger age groups—and the variability of their absorption and metabolism in adults—careful monitoring of adverse side effects is necessary when these medications are used with children and adolescents.

Clinical Effects

There is limited research describing the clinical effects of the antipsychotic medications on children and adolescents. As a result, approaches to their use with pediatric populations often are based on clinical trials that were conducted on adults. In general, the antipsychotic medications appear to be effective in reducing hallucinations, delusions, ideas of reference, and the formal thought disorder experienced by adults with schizophrenia. The drugs appear less effective in addressing problems such as withdrawal, flattening of affect, amotivation, and apathy. The high-potency medications are generally preferred for the treatment of children and adolescents because they are less sedating. The limited research that has been conducted with children and adolescents has focused largely on the effectiveness of haloperidol to reduce the symptoms of childhood schizophrenia (M. Campbell et al.,1993; E. K. Spencer et al.,1992). There also is evidence that haloperidol can reduce a number of the problematic behaviors exhibited by children with autism (M. Campbell & Cueva, 1995a, 1995b), and that it is effective in reducing the motor and vocal tics associated with Tourette's disorder.

In clinical practice, antipsychotic medications are also sometimes used to manage disruptive behaviors exhibited by children and adolescents. There is some evidence to support the use of haloperidol with children who exhibit explosive aggressiveness and with autistic children who show aggressive behavior (M. Campbell et al., 1993). However, there is little evidence supporting the effectiveness of antipsychotic medications for children with more general disruptive behavior. Further, the drugs have potential adverse side effects on children's cognitive and learning abilities. Thus, physicians should be cautious in prescribing antipsychotic medications to manage children whose problems are limited primarily to disruptive or oppositional behavior. This need for caution can create difficulties for physicians who may be subjected to considerable pressure to do something to reduce the disruptive behavior of children at school.

Because environmental events often maintain self-injurious behaviors, a more effective approach might combine antipsychotic agents with behavior management. M. Campbell, Anderson, et al. (1978) compared behavior therapy, haloperidol, and their combination in a study of 40 preschool children diagnosed with autism. The combination of drug therapy and behavior therapy was found to be superior to either treatment alone, particularly for language acquisition. Similarly, the combination of therapies was found to be more effective than either medication or behavior therapy for stereotypies and withdrawn behavior.

Specific psychiatric disorders are more frequently found in children and adolescents with mental retardation than in children of normal intelligence (M. Campbell & Malone, 1991; M. Campbell et al., 1993). When behavioral interventions do not prove successful for severe aggression, overactivity, and self-injurious behavior, antipsychotic agents may be used. Although a number of investigations have evaluated various psychotropic agents in mentally retarded children and adolescents (for review, see Aman & Singh, 1988, 1991; Gadow & Poling, 1988; Poling et al., 1991b), the results are difficult to interpret because of methodological difficulties, diagnostic vagueness, and small sample sizes (M. Campbell et al., 1993).

In recent years, a great deal of legislation has addressed the appropriate treatment of the mentally retarded in residential treatment centers (Gadow & Poling, 1988). In those settings, it is imperative to use only appropriate pharmacotherapies that meet the rigorous standards of carefully controlled trials to validate the efficacy and safety of these medications for the mentally retarded. Finally, studies are needed that investigate the effects of antipsychotic medications on cognition and adaptive behavioral functioning in children and adolescents with mental retardation (Aman, 1984).

Adverse Side Effects and Toxicity

The antipsychotic medications have a number of severe adverse side effects which in some cases may be irreversible (M. A. Richardson et al., 1991). It is essential that school staff responsible for the care of children receiving antipsychotic medication be familiar with these adverse side effects. Children's physicians must be consulted immediately if children receiving antipsychotic medications experience adverse side effects. This is particularly important if a child appears to be experiencing any of the neurological effects described in Table 5.5.

Adverse neurological effects may be classified according to the part of the body they affect or whether they occur in the short term or are idiosyncratic. Table 5.5 also presents those adverse side effects and reactions to antipsychotic medications.

Important adverse neurological effects that may occur in children and adolescents are termed *extrapyramidal symptoms*. Adolescents appear particularly sensitive to these symptoms, which can be divided into four types: acute dystonic reactions, Parkinsonian symptoms, akathisia, and akinesia.

Acute dystonic reactions usually develop very soon after children commence treatment. They may manifest as a twisting of a child's neck to one side (torticollis) or a dramatic rolling back of a child's eyes under the eyelids (oculogyric crisis). These symptoms may be rapidly relieved with anticholinergic medications such as benzotropine or diphenhydramine ad-

TABLE 5.5. Untoward Effects of Antipsychotic Medications

Short-term	Long-term	Idiosyncratic
Acute dystonia	Hepatic toxicity	Agranulocytosis
Affective blunting	Hyperprolactinemia	Neuroleptic malignant
Akathisia	Ocular pigmentation	syndrome
Anticholinergic symptoms	Tardive dyskinesia	Sudden death
Cardiac arrhythmias		
Cognitive dulling		
Extrapyramidal symptoms		
Sedation		
Social withdrawal		

Note. Adapted from Rosenberg et al. (1994). Copyright 1994 by Taylor & Francis. Adapted by permission.

ministered orally or intramuscularly. The experience of acute dystonia can be very frightening for children and adolescents. If they are not forewarned about its possible occurrence, parents and children may also lose faith in the treatment. Families must be informed about this potential problem and the steps to treat it quickly. School staff responsible for children who commence treatment with antipsychotic medication also must know the steps to treat this adverse side effect.

Parkinsonian symptoms may occur within the first 2–3 weeks of commencing treatment with an antipsychotic medication. The effects include a fixed facial expression, a lack of arm swinging when walking, a hand tremor, and a rigidity in the limbs. In general, this adverse side effect is treated by reducing the amount of medication. Akathisia usually occurs within the first few months of treatment. It is characterized by motor restlessness, with children or adolescents appearing very agitated and reporting that they feel driven. Assessment of akathisia can be difficult because it can be confused with increased anxiety or agitation arising as a result of a child's underlying disorder. Akinesia is characterized by a lack of gestures, spontaneity, emotions, and speech. Awareness of these signs is important to avoid mistaking them for the onset of a depressive disorder.

The most important long-term adverse side effects are various abnormal involuntary movements (dyskinesias). These movements may involve the muscles of any part of the body but most frequently affect muscles of the mouth, face, tongue, jaws, or limbs. The nature of the involuntary movements varies but often involves slow, rhythmical movements of the affected muscle groups. The movements associated with chronic administration of antipsychotic medication are known as tardive dyskinesia, and movements that arise when the dosage is reduced or discontinued are called withdrawal dyskinesias. McClellan and Werry (1994) suggest that withdrawal dyskinesias almost always resolve over time, but tardive dyskinesia may continue even after the antipsychotic drug is discontinued. There is no proven treatment for tardive dyskinesia. It is important for parents and children to understand the nature of these dyskinesias and for physicians to use the minimum effective doses of medication when treating children. Chapter 4 presents a more extended discussion of tardive dyskinesia.

Children and adolescents who receive antipsychotic medications may experience a range of other adverse side effects reflecting the broad types of actions of antipsychotic medications (Table 5.5). Sedation and weight gain are two adverse side effects that are particularly upsetting for children and adolescents. The former can interfere with children's learning, and the latter is distressing for adolescents who are sensitive to their body image. Antipsychotic medications can also lower the seizure threshold. As a result, caution is necessary when prescribing antipsychotic medication for children with a seizure disorder or for children who are at risk of developing seizures, such as children with autism or brain damage.

Two other severe adverse side effects should be noted. The first is neuroleptic malignant syndrome, which is a rare but potentially life-threatening effect of antipsychotic medications. The syndrome is characterized by hyperthermia, "lead pipe" muscular rigidity, altered mental status, rapid heart rate, and pallor. Its onset should be treated as an emergency requiring immediate medical treatment. The second adverse side effect is a blood dyscrasia, agranulocytosis, that is potentially fatal and that can arise during treatment with the new antipsychotic medication clozapine. Thus, it is important that children being treated with clozapine have regular blood monitoring.

Dosage and Administration

Antipsychotic medications are almost invariably administered orally to children, and the dosages of different antipsychotics vary greatly (Werry & Aman, 1993b). There is little evidence of the superiority of individual antipsychotics for the treatment of schizophrenia (McClellan & Werry, 1994). As a result, the choice of medication typically is based on the history of medication response, the antidopaminergic potency of the drug, and the risk of adverse side effects of the medication. McClellan and Werry noted that antipsychotics have not been studied in the younger age groups and suggested that their use should be restricted to adolescents with schizophrenia who have a history of chronic symptoms and poor compliance with medication.

Approaches to medication use tend to vary in different situations. For children or adolescents who are admitted to the hospital with florid symptoms of schizophrenia, somewhat higher dosages of antipsychotic medication are employed. Initially, the effect of the antipsychotic medications is largely sedative, with the antipsychotic effects only becoming evident after 1 to 2 weeks (McClellan & Werry, 1994). Subsequently, maintenance doses of medication are used to stop relapses. In contrast, children whose initial illness is less severe may be initially treated with lower dosages. Adjustments are then made to the dosage until an effective level is identified.

The use of prophylactic anti-Parkinsonian drugs is controversial. McClellan and Werry (1994) suggest that prophylactic use of these drugs should be restricted to children or adolescents who are at high risk for acute dystonias (e.g., adolescent males), children receiving high dosages of medication, or children with a history of dystonias. Furthermore, they suggest that attempts should be made to discontinue anti-Parkinsonian drugs after 2–3 months because two thirds of children will no longer need them after this time. As noted earlier, if prophylactic anti-Parkinsonian drugs are not employed, children, parents, and teachers must be advised of the appropriate steps to take if a child suffers an acute dystonia. The key principle for prescribing antipsychotic medication is to maintain children on the lowest effective dose to minimize the risk of adverse neurological effects, particularly tardive dyskinesia. Physicians employ several techniques to achieve this aim. These include regular attempts during the maintenance phase of treatment to lower the medication dosage and reviews every 6 months to assess the need to continue medication (McClellan & Werry, 1994). Observations by school staff can help identify the minimum effective dosage of antipsychotic medication, and staff can monitor children for the presence of adverse neurological effects. It is beyond the scope of this chapter to provide guidelines for dosages of all the available antipsychotic medications; however, an overview of dosage levels is provided in several pharmacology texts (Rosenberg et al., 1994; Werry & Aman, 1993b).

Summary

The antipsychotic medications (or neuroleptics) are considered to be the treatment of choice for managing schizophrenia in children and adolescents. In some circumstances they may also be helpful in the management of other psychiatric disorders in children and adolescents, including, autism, conduct disorder, ADHD with aggression, and Tourette's disorder.

The host of adverse effects associated with the neuroleptics, including extrapyramidal symptoms, dyskinesias, lethargy, and weight gain, mandate their careful and judicious use in pediatric populations. They are generally safest when used at the lowest possible doses. The most pervasive short-term adverse effect of antipsychotics is cognitive impairment that may result in learning and academic difficulties. Some research suggests that cognitive and behavioral toxicities are dose dependent, with lower doses reducing the impact of these adverse effects. Despite these toxicities, when judiciously prescribed and appropriately monitored, the therapeutic effects of antipsychotics for children with symptoms of psychosis and/or aggression can be striking, allowing severely disturbed children and adolescents to remain at home with their families and in special education classrooms in lieu of residential treatment centers.

Tricyclics, Selective Serotonin Reuptake Inhibitors, and Monoamine Oxidase Inhibitors

The drugs discussed in this section are presented in Table 5.6. They are traditionally grouped together because they are employed to treat depressive disorders in adults. However, the term *antidepressants* is inappropriate

TABLE 5.6. Heterocyclic Antidepressants

Generic name	Trade name
Tertiary amines	
Amitriptyline	Elavil, Endep
Clomipramine	Anafranil
Doxepin	Sinequan, Adapin
Imipramine	Tofranil
Secondary amines	
Desipramine	Norpramin, Pertofrane
Nortriptyline	Pamelor, Arentyl
Protriptyline	Vivactil, Concordin
Trimipramine	Surmontil
Dibenzoxazepines	
Amoxapine	Asendin
Tetracyclics	
Maprotiline	Ludiomil
Triazolopyridines	
Trazodone	Desyrel
Benzenepropanamines	
Fluoxetine	Prozac
Propiophenones	
Buproprion	Wellbutrin

Note. From Werry & Aman (1993a). Copyright 1993 by Plenum Publishing Corp. Reprinted by permission.

to describe their use with children because there is little evidence that they are an effective treatment for depressive disorders experienced by children and adolescents.

The tricyclic medications and the monoamine oxidase inhibitors (MAOIs) were first identified more than 40 years ago. The MAOIs were used to treat tuberculosis before anyone recognized their mood-elevating properties. For many years the treatment of adult depressive disorders relied heavily on the use of tricyclic medications; MAOIs were employed when patients had a poor response to tricyclics. The SSRIs are an important new group of medications that are widely used with adults. Advantages of the SSRIs include their lack of cholinergic side effects, lower risk of cardiac side effects, and fewer withdrawal symptoms. To date, however, few studies describe the effectiveness of SSRIs in managing childhood and adolescent psychiatric disorders. Nevertheless, SSRIs are increasingly being used to manage a range of childhood and adolescent mental disorders.

Although tricyclic medications traditionally have been employed to treat symptoms associated with depression in adults, the parameters of antidepressant medication have been expanded more recently to include not only major depressive disorder and dysthymia (for review, see Ambrosini et al., 1993a; Ambrosini, Bianchi, Rabinovich, & Elia, 1993b; Pliszka, 1991; Steingard, DeMaso, Goldman, Shorrock, & Bucci, 1995), but also many other psychiatric disorders in children and adolescents. Tricyclics are now used to manage several other childhood disorders such as ADHD (Biederman, Baldessarini, Wright, Knee, & Harmatz, 1989; Rapoport et al., 1974), separation anxiety disorder in school phobia (Gittelman-Klein & Klein, 1971, 1973), overanxious disorder (Birmaher et al., 1994), obsessive–compulsive disorder (DeVeaugh-Geiss et al., 1992; Flament et al., 1985; Liebowitz et al., 1990), enuresis (Blackwell & Currah, 1973), sleep disorders (Pliszka, 1991), and bulimia (Fava et al., 1990; Pope, Hudson, Jonas, & Yurgelun-Todd, 1983).

Management of ADHD using tricyclics was reported in the 1970s (Waizer, Hoffman, Pulizos, & Englehardt, 1974), but studies comparing the effectiveness of tricyclics with the stimulants found stimulants to be superior for the management of ADHD-related symptoms (Garfinkel, Wender, Sloman, & O'Neill, 1983; Rapoport et al., 1974). The tricyclics are most beneficial for children with ADHD who have comorbid mood and anxiety disorders (Pliszka, 1991; T. Spencer, Biederman, Kerman, Steingard, & Wilens, 1993).

Holttum, Lubetsky, and Eastman (1994) described a case study of an autistic girl with trichotillomania (hair pulling) who was treated with both tricyclic medication and behavioral therapy. Although neither treatment alone helped reduce symptoms, the combination of the two treatments was effective in managing the behavior. Approximately 3 months after cessation of treatment, however, symptoms of anxiety and hair pulling returned to pretreatment levels.

Clomipramine reduces many of the symptoms experienced by children and adolescents with obsessive-compulsive disorder (DeVeaugh-Geiss et al., 1992; Flament et al., 1985; Leonard et al., 1989). Gittelman-Klein and Klein (1971) reported that tricyclics reduce separation anxiety (commonly present in children experiencing school phobia), but more recent investigations did not replicate their findings (Bernstein et al., 1990).

Pharmacology and Pharmacokinetics

The actions of this group of medications are largely mediated through their effect on neurotransmitters, especially norepinephrine and serotonin (Hardman et al., 1996). In general, the tricyclic medications and SSRIs potentiate the actions of these neurotransmitters by blocking their reuptake into the synapses, thus prolonging their action in the synaptic cleft.

Tricyclics and SSRIs vary in the extent to which they block different neurotransmitters. The SSRIs have a relatively selective effect on serotonin, whereas the tricyclic medications generally block norepinephrine, with a more limited effect on serotonin.

The MAOIs affect a large range of systems within the body. However, their effect on psychiatric disorders primarily reflects their ability to reduce the speed with which monoamine neurotransmitters are degraded by monoamine oxidases. These actions increase the availability of neurotransmitters in the synaptic cleft.

Children and adolescents metabolize these medications more rapidly than do adults. In addition, blood levels achieved with the same oral dosage may vary greatly with children and adolescents. As a result, the effects of different dosage levels must be monitored carefully for children who take these medications. The tricyclic drugs have a relatively long half-life, and it is theoretically possible to administer only one dose a day for adults. However, with children, two doses daily are recommended to avoid the possibility of withdrawal effects because children rapidly metabolize the medication. To help ensure that children receive the most effective dosage to treat their disorder, blood levels of some of these medications can be monitored.

Clinical Effects

The tricyclic medications are used primarily to treat four mental disorders experienced by children and adolescents: depressive disorders, ADHD, anxiety disorders, and enuresis (bed wetting). However, although the tricyclics are widely used to treat childhood depressive disorders, there is no evidence to that they are more effective than placebo for managing children's depressive disorders (Ambrosini et al., 1993a; R. L. Fisher & Fisher, 1996; B. Geller et al., 1992; Hazell, O'Connell, Heathcote, Robertson, & Henry, 1995; Kutcher et al., 1994).

The advent of the SSRIs has significantly affected the treatment of depressive disorders experienced by adults, with one member of the group, fluoxetine (Prozac) becoming the subject of considerable media interest. DeVane and Sallee (1996) reviewed the published clinical and research literature on SSRIs in children and adolescents. Their review on the use of SSRIs in pediatric samples included 16 open trials, 3 double-blind trials, and 23 case studies. These investigations studied a combined total of more than 400 patients. The review concluded that evidence exists for use of SSRIs in the treatment of depression and obsessive–compulsive disorder in adolescents.

The longest period of long-term follow-up with an SSRI in the research was 19 months and involved the use of fluoxetine for obsessive–

compulsive disorder (D. A. Geller et al., 1995). The investigators reported marked to moderate global symptom improvement in nearly three-quarters of the 38 children and adolescents who participated in the study. The authors interpreted their findings as suggesting that fluoxetine may be effective in prepubertal children and that, more important, this effect can be sustained over a relatively long period with few adverse side effects. Similarly, a 2-year follow-up investigation of children treated with tricyclic antidepressant medication found that the medication reduced obsessive–compulsive symptoms in the majority of cases.

In a similar study, Birmaher et al. (1994) examined the efficacy of fluoxetine for the management of 21 children and adolescents with anxiety disorders, including overanxious disorder, social phobia, and separation anxiety disorder, that were unresponsive to other pharmacological and psychotherapeutic interventions. The children were treated for up to 10 months, and most of those who received fluoxetine showed moderate to marked improvement. The authors interpreted the data as supporting fluoxetine's effectiveness and safety for the management of anxiety disorders in children and adolescents. Unfortunately, no additional follow-up was conducted, thus limiting our knowledge about the long-term efficacy and potential adverse late effects.

In one of the few studies of the longer-term effect of SSRIs, Cook et al. (1992) conducted an open trial of fluoxetine with children and adults with autistic disorder and mental retardation. The length of treatment ranged from 6 months to over 1 year. The majority of children were rated as improved, although many of the subjects experienced significant adverse side effects that impeded their daily functioning.

All the follow-up studies conducted on SSRIs and the treatment of depression were conducted over a 2-month period (Apter et al., 1994; Boulos, Kutcher, Gardner, & Young, 1992; Jain et al., 1992; Simeon, Dinicola, Ferguson, & Copping, 1990), with no reported follow-up studies beyond that period. As SSRIs have only recently come into use as a pharmacotherapy for children, studies of their long-term effects are in their infancy. This is an important area for future research.

There is some evidence to suggest that although less effective than the stimulants, the tricyclics are more effective than placebo for treating symptoms associated with ADHD (Biederman, Baldessarini, Wright, Keenan, & Faraone, 1993; Biederman et al., 1989; Pliszka, 1987). These empirical data encouraged physicians to use tricyclic medications as alternatives to stimulants to manage ADHD when children do not show an adequate response to stimulant medication (Ambrosini et al., 1993b). One medication in this group, clomipramine, also appears to be particularly effective for treating obsessive–compulsive disorder (DeVeaugh-Geiss et al., 1992; Piccinelli, Pini, Bellantuono, & Wilkinson, 1995). Evidence also suggests that SSRIs may help reduce symptoms of obsessive–compulsive disorder experienced by children and adolescents (Ambrosini et al., 1993b; Geller et al., 1995; Piccinelli et al., 1995; M. A. Riddle et al., 1992). The effectiveness of the tricyclic medications for the management of the other anxiety disorders is less clear. Although an early study suggested that imipramine was effective in treating separation anxiety disorder, a later replication reported that imipramine was no more effective than placebo (Klein, Koplewicz, & Kanner, 1992).

Although tricyclic medications can effectively stop bed wetting in the short term, Viesselman et al. (1993) suggested that children commonly develop tolerance, and enuresis often resumes when medication is stopped. In light of this, behavioral techniques are the preferred treatment for children with enuresis. Use of tricyclic medications should be limited to situations in which immediate cessation is required for short periods, for example, when children attend overnight summer camp.

The role of the MAOIs for the management of childhood disorders appears quite limited. Their use should only be considered in controlled situations such as inpatient wards when all other treatments have failed.

Adverse Side Effects and Toxicity

Anticholinergic adverse side effects associated with tricyclic medications include dry mouth, constipation, nausea, tiredness, blurred vision, and urinary retention. Sedation also is a common adverse side effect of many tricyclic medications, and this may be a disadvantage for schoolchildren. Further, a small number of children receiving tricyclic medications experience seizures, and children with a previous history of seizures may be at greater risk for this adverse side effect.

Tricyclic medications have a major effect on the cardiovascular system, and there are reports of sudden deaths among children taking desipramine (Leonard et al., 1995). Although the medication's role in these deaths remains unclear, the reports underscore the need for caution when tricyclic medications are being used to treat children and adolescents (M. A. Riddle, Geller, & Ryan, 1993). The reports also emphasize the importance of carefully assessing children's cardiac status before commencing tricyclic medications and carefully monitoring children during the time they receive the medications. It also is extremely important to be aware that if a child takes an overdose of tricyclic medications, the effects of the medication on the cardiovascular system may be life threatening. Any child who takes an overdose of tricyclic medications should be assessed by a physician immediately, followed by careful cardiac and respiratory monitoring.

When tricyclic medications are withdrawn, some children experience a flu-like withdrawal syndrome, with symptoms such as nausea, abdominal discomfort, headache, and fatigue. If these symptoms are severe, tricyclic medication can be reintroduced and then gradually tapered to minimize the withdrawal symptoms. As noted, children who rapidly metabolize the drugs may experience these symptoms even though they continue to receive the medication.

The SSRIs have a range of adverse side effects on the gastrointestinal system, including nausea, diarrhea, dyspepsia, and weight loss. Adverse behavioral effects include motor restlessness, social disinhibition, and sleep difficulty (Ambrosini et al., 1993b). As noted by Ambrosini et al. (1993b), the SSRIs can also interact with a range of other medications employed to treat childhood psychiatric disorders. As a result, physicians should take great care when they prescribe SSRIs for patients who are taking other medications. One study suggested that adults receiving fluoxetine may develop suicidal preoccupation (Teicher, Glod, & Cole, 1990). Although there is limited evidence of this occurring among children and adolescents, King et al. (1991) identified several possible reasons for the emergence of suicidal thoughts among children receiving SSRIs. These reasons include the possibility that the suicidal thoughts may arise coincidentally to treatment with fluoxetine, they may emerge as part of medication-induced mood changes, or they may be a specific effect of the medication.

The MAOIs can cause severe adverse side effects. In particular, a hypertensive crisis can occur if substances containing tyramine are ingested while children are receiving MAOIs. It is important that children and parents be aware of this effect and know that the children must avoid foods containing tyramine, including cheese, broad beans, and chocolate. Careful monitoring of the diet of schoolchildren is difficult, and school staff should obtain advice from a dietician about the full range of foods to be avoided. In addition, severe illness including confusion, fever, agitation, and seizures can occur if SSRIs are prescribed at the same time as MAOIs. As a result, children should not be treated with this combination of medications.

Dosage and Administration

A number of psychopharmacology texts can be consulted to obtain dosage information about medications in this group. (Green 1995; Rosenberg et al., 1994; Werry & Aman, 1993b). However, readers should note that in contrast to the rapid action of some of the other medications described in this chapter, tricyclic medications or SSRIs may take several weeks to achieve therapeutic effects. As a result, the dose of tricyclic medications or SSRIs should not be increased rapidly if they initially appear to have little effect on children's symptoms.

Finally, the tricyclic medications must be administered carefully because overdosage can have severe adverse effects, including death. Children must be carefully supervised while they receive the medication. At all times, medications must be stored securely at home and at school. In particular, medication should be inaccessible to adolescents with suicidal ideation. The correct dosage must be given to children and adolescents, and proper treatment must be obtained rapidly if children show evidence of adverse side effects.

Summary

For children and adolescents, the tricyclics have been employed primarily to manage symptoms associated with ADHD, depressive disorders, anxiety disorders, and enuresis. Although there is some support for their role in managing symptoms associated with ADHD, there is little evidence that tricyclics are effective for treating depression in pediatric populations. In recent years, SSRIs increasingly have been used to manage various psychiatric disorders in children, although empirical support is lacking for the drugs' clinical efficacy. The primary adverse side effects of the tricyclics are cardiovascular toxicities, and they are potentially lethal in large doses. For this reason, the administration of tricyclics must be carefully managed. Although the SSRIs offer the advantage of a potentially safer side effect profile, further clinical trials are needed before endorsing their efficacy in pediatric populations.

Lithium

Lithium is a naturally occurring alkaline metal that is widely used to treat manic episodes in adults with bipolar disorders and as maintenance therapy for bipolar patients with a history of mania. Lithium's effectiveness for the treatment of mania was first reported in 1949 by Cade in Australia. Alessi et al. (1994) recently highlighted the impact of this drug on the treatment of bipolar illness; they reported that more than 16,000 articles about lithium were published since its discovery, with more than 1,000 articles added annually. However, Alessi et al. (1994) point out that only 58 of these articles described the use of lithium with children and adolescents. As noted elsewhere in this chapter, the vast literature describing the effectiveness of psychotropic drugs for adults with mental disorders, combined with the paucity of studies describing their effectiveness with children and adolescents, creates a dilemma for physicians who must decide whether a psychotropic medication should be used to treat children or adolescents experiencing psychiatric disorders.

Pharmacology and Pharmacokinetics

Although a wide range of lithium's actions have been described, the exact mechanism by which it exerts its psychotropic effects remains unclear (Alessi et al., 1994; Hardman et al., 1996). Lithium is rapidly absorbed from the gastrointestinal tract and reaches peak blood levels in 2–4 hours after administration of the oral dose. Approximately 90% of a dose of lithium is eliminated through the kidneys, and there is a close relationship between lithium and sodium excretion by the kidneys. As a result, children who develop abnormalities in their sodium balance (e.g., by becoming severely dehydrated or by using salt-free diets) are at risk for developing lithium toxicity.

Clinical Effects

In a recent review, Alessi et al. (1994) suggested that lithium should be considered for the management of aggression and bipolar illness among children and adolescents. However, bipolar illness is rare among children, and few studies describe the effectiveness of lithium to treat childhood bipolar illness (Viesselman et al., 1993). As a result, physicians must extrapolate from results in adult studies when they consider whether to use lithium to treat children. Not surprisingly, this leads physicians to use lithium to treat children with disorders that appear similar to bipolar disorders experienced by adults.

Alessi et al. (1994) reported that, for adults, aggression "continues to be the most widely supported clinical diagnostic entity for which lithium is indicated" (p. 293). However, few studies support the effectiveness of lithium to reduce aggression in children, and the few investigations that were conducted largely focused on institutionalized children or adolescents (Alessi et al., 1994; M. Campbell, Small, et al., 1984; Viesselman et al., 1993). Therefore, caution is warranted in the use of lithium to manage childhood and adolescent aggression, and careful monitoring of the beneficial and adverse side effects of the drug is essential.

Adverse Side Effects and Toxicity

Adverse side effects of lithium are common and quickly occur if blood levels increase beyond the treatment range. To avoid such adverse side effects, blood lithium levels must be monitored regularly during treatment, and dosages need to be adjusted to maintain blood levels within the therapeutic range.

Adverse side effects of lithium include a fine tremor, abdominal discomfort, excessive drinking and urination, and weight gain. For adolescents, an important adverse side effect is the onset or exacerbation of acne. The onset of lithium toxicity is characterized by vomiting, profuse diarrhea, coarse tremor, coma, or convulsions. If these symptoms are observed in a child receiving lithium, immediate medical treatment should be initiated. Lithium also can cause birth defects in a fetus. In light of this, clinicians should carefully consider the likelihood of adolescents becoming pregnant while they are being treated with lithium.

Dosage and Administration

Appropriate lithium dosage is determined by monitoring lithium blood levels. The aim of this monitoring is to achieve a therapeutic steady-state blood level of lithium in the range 0.6–1.2mEq/liter (Alessi et al., 1994). Recently, Green (1995) suggested that children's lithium levels may be monitored through saliva tests to avoid the need for repeated and potentially upsetting blood tests. However, Alessi et al. (1994) point out that saliva sampling has limitations, including the requirement that children must not eat or drink for 12 hours before samples are taken.

Summary

Although much research attests to the efficacy of lithium for adults, few data are available to guide the clinical use of lithium for children and adolescents. Some research suggests that lithium is effective for children and adolescents exhibiting aggression. However, these studies were conducted primarily in residential treatment centers and inpatient hospital facilities. Ongoing monitoring of lithium levels is necessary, and their potential adverse side effects may be toxic. For this reason, judicious use and ongoing monitoring is imperative for pediatric populations.

Antiepileptic Medications

Carbamazepine and valproate are two antiepileptic drugs that may, at times, be used to manage child or adolescent psychiatric disorders. Carbamazepine is an antiepileptic medication chemically related to the tricyclic medications. It also is effective for the treatment of trigeminal glossopharyngeal neuralgias. Valproate is a medication that is effective in the treatment of epilepsy.

Pharmacology and Pharmacokinetics

The pharmacokinetic characteristics of carbamazepine are complex. It is absorbed slowly and erratically after oral administration. Although peak

blood levels may be achieved approximately 4 to 8 hours after oral ingestion, they may be delayed for longer periods (Hardman et al., 1996). Valproate is absorbed rapidly after oral administration. Peak blood levels are
achieved within 1 to 4 hours with a half-life of approximately 15 hours.

Clinical Effects

The principal use of carbamazepine and valproate is for the treatment of
seizures. However, carbamazepine is used to manage various mental disorders in adults, particularly mania, when lithium is ineffective. It is important to note, however, that there are no double-blind trials of its effectiveness to treat childhood disorders. With children, both carbamazepine
and valproate tend to be employed when other medications are ineffective
in the management of severe childhood disorders. However, Viesselman
et al. (1993) emphasized the lack of studies investigating the effectiveness
of valproate and suggest that it should be treated as experimental in the
context of treating child psychiatric disorders.

Adverse Side Effects and Toxicity

The frequent use of carbamazepine and valproate to treat seizures experienced by children and adolescents means that considerable information is
available about their adverse side effects (Carpenter & Vining, 1993). Approximately one-third of patients who are treated with carbamazepine experience some unwanted effects, including nausea, drowsiness, dizziness,
ataxia, blurred vision, and diplopia (Waters, 1990). In addition, children
may experience a leukopenia and a maculopapular rash.

Valproate can cause severe liver damage, so it should not be administered to children with a history of liver disease. Other adverse side effects
include sedation, nausea, vomiting, and indigestion. Valproate also can result in marked elevation of the blood levels of other anticonvulsant medications. For example, Hardman et al. (1996) reported that the concentration of phenobarbital may rise by as much as 40% when administered in
concert with valproate.

Summary

The antiepileptics are sometimes employed to manage psychiatric disorders in children and adolescents when other psychopharmacological
agents fail. However, there is little systematic empirical investigation of
these agents for the management of various pediatric psychiatric disorders. Because of the widespread use of the antiepileptics in managing
seizure disorders in children and adolescents, much is known about their

adverse side effects that affect approximately one third of the pediatric population receiving these agents. Certainly, greater research efforts are needed to evaluate the efficacy of the antiepileptics in managing psychiatric disorders in children and adolescents. Until these data are forthcoming, judicious use of these medications in managing mental disorders in pediatric groups is recommended.

Hypnotics and Sedatives

A sedative medication is defined as a medication that decreases activity, moderates excitement, and calms the recipients. A hypnotic medication produces drowsiness and facilitates the onset and maintenance of a state of sleep that resembles natural sleep (Hardman et al., 1996). The widespread use of these medications in primary health care is a reflection of their low toxicity, ease of use, and effectiveness in the short-term reduction of anxiety and insomnia experienced by adults.

The value of hypnotics and sedatives for treating childhood psychiatric disorders appears limited, with several reviews highlighting the paucity of evidence demonstrating the effectiveness of these medications in treating anxiety disorders experienced by children or adolescents (Gadow, 1992; Rosenberg et al., 1994; Werry & Aman, 1993b). Despite this paucity of evidence, the medications are widely prescribed for children and adolescents in the community. For example, hypnotic drugs are commonly prescribed for childhood insomnia, although some suggest that most of these prescriptions are not justified and the benefits of sedatives used with children have yet to be established (Rosenberg et al., 1994; Werry & Aman, 1993b).

Pharmacology and Pharmacokinetics

There are three main groups of hypnotic–sedative medications: the benzodiazepines, the antihistamines, and a third, somewhat heterogeneous, group of medications. The benzodiazepines are rapidly absorbed via oral or parenteral routes and are categorized as short, intermediate, or long acting, or as high- or low-potency drugs (Werry & Aman, 1993b). The clinical benefits of benzodiazepines are due to their effect on the CNS, primarily their influence on the inhibitory neurotransmitter receptor system activated by GABA (Hardman et al., 1996). The second group of sedative and hypnotic medications is the antihistamines (e.g., diphenhydramine, promethazine), widely used to manage sleeping problems in young children. These drugs appear to produce sedation by blocking the H_1 histamine receptor system. This is one of the three receptor systems through which histamine exerts its effect, and antihistamines developed to act primarily on other histamine receptor systems do not seem to have a sedative effect.

The third group of drugs includes a range of other medications, such as the barbiturates that were used in the past for sedation or the treatment of anxiety. Problems with physical dependence, tolerance, and severe withdrawal reactions led to the replacement of the barbiturates with other medications. Another member of this group, buspirone, attracted interest because of its anxiolytic properties with adults. Buspirone is one of a new class of medications called azapirones that have a particular affinity for serotonin receptors. This medication appears to cause less sedation than other medications used for the treatment of anxiety, and it may be less likely to cause medication dependence.

Clinical Effects

Werry and Aman suggested (1993b) that the effects of the benzodiazepines resemble the effects of alcohol. Furthermore, these authors suggest that some of the paradoxical effects of the benzodiazepines for children can be explained as an interaction between the direct effects of the medication, the social setting in which the medication is used, and the mood state of the individual using the medication. Thus, they suggest that in quiet states, sleep is likely to intervene, whereas in group situations uninhibited behavior or hostility may occur, depending on the group setting. Werry and Aman noted that the paradoxical effect of benzodiazepines that was described with children may reflect the social context in which the medications are used. For example, an agitated and anxious child who is given medication in a stressful and upsetting situation may well become more upset and irritable rather than becoming more settled.

As noted, there is little evidence that the benzodiazepines are effective for the management of anxiety disorders experienced by children. Despite this, the benzodiazepines are widely used to manage childhood anxiety disorders and Waters (1990) suggested that current usage far exceeds any effectiveness supported by evidence in the literature. Werry and Aman (1993) also pointed out that much of the support for prescribing these medications to children is based on studies of adults. However, it is difficult to extrapolate from adult studies because the anxiety disorders experienced by children often differ from those of adults.

The clinical literature does suggest that both alprazolam and clonazepam may be effective in the management of panic disorder (Biederman, 1987; M. Campbell & Cueva, 1995a, 1995b; Kutcher & MacKenzie, 1988). Ross and Piggott (1993) reported the viability of clonazepam for a 14-year-old male who was hospitalized for a severely disabling obsessive–compulsive disorder. However, few controlled trials with these agents were reported in the literature. Graae et al. (1994) investigated the efficacy of clonazepam in a double-blind, placebo-controlled crossover study in 15 children with anxiety disorders. The majority of subjects demonstrated moderate to marked clinical improvement, and 50% of the children no longer met diagnostic criteria for anxiety disorder at the end of the study. However, the overall changes did not reach statistical significance, possibly due to the small number of subjects. Adverse side effects included lethargy, lability, and disinhibition (e.g., irritability, tantrums, and aggressivity). Thus, although clonazepam shows potential promise in the management of anxiety disorders in children, additional studies are warranted, particularly research that systematically examines the adverse side effects of this medication in the context of its influences on learning and behavior.

In a double-blind placebo-controlled study, Lucas and Pasley (1969) evaluated the efficacy of a 16-week course of diazepam for subjects who ranged from 7 to 17 years. Target symptoms included levels of anxiety, oppositional behavior, poor peer relationships, and aggression. No significant differences were found between diazepam and placebo for the individual target behaviors. The authors concluded that diazepam was not clinically effective in reducing anxiety or acting-out behavior in children and adolescents.

The antihistamines have been used for many years to sedate young children with disturbed sleep. However, there is limited evidence to support the drugs' effectiveness, and it appears the problem often recurs when the medication is discontinued (Richman, Douglas, Hunt, Lansdown, & Levere, 1985). If antihistamines are used for sedation, they should only be used for short periods during which appropriate behavioral interventions are initiated. Rosenberg et al. (1994) also suggested caution in using benzodiazepines to treat insomnia. In many cases the half-life of the benzodiazepines is long, and residual daytime effects may linger if the medication is used to improve sleep at night. In addition, rebound insomnia may occur after prolonged usage of benzodiazepines for the purpose of improving sleep.

Adverse Side Effects and Toxicity

A lack of toxicity is one of the attractive features of this group of medications; however, sedation at higher dosages and behavioral disinhibition in some social settings are potential problems. Care must be taken when prescribing these medications for adolescents because of the potential for abuse and the risk of causing impaired driving, particularly if adolescents are also using alcohol. For children at school, important adverse side effects include possible memory impairment, impairment of other cognitive functions, reduction in sustained attention, and motor incoordination.

Other adverse side effects of antihistamines include dizziness, sedation, agitation, abdominal pain, blurred vision, and dry mouth (R. T. Brown & Dingle, 1994).

Dosage and Administration

There have been few clinical trials to identify the appropriate dosage levels of sedatives and hypnotics for children and adolescents. In general, the minimum effective dosage should be employed, the need for the medication should be reviewed regularly, and medication should be discontinued within a few weeks.

If benzodiazepines have been used over a prolonged period, a gradual tapering of the dosage is necessary when the medications are to be discontinued. Otherwise children may have withdrawal symptoms, including insomnia, anxiety, tremulousness, and irritability. These symptoms may be a particular problem if benzodiazepines have been used to manage a sleep disorder. In this situation, symptoms of rebound insomnia may lead naive users of the medication to recommence their use because they believe they have suffered a relapse of the original sleep disorder.

Summary

Despite the widespread clinical use of the hypnotics and sedatives in managing various sleep-related and anxiety disorders in children and adolescents, there are limited data available to support the efficacy of these medications. Sedation and behavioral disinhibition are common adverse side effects, and these effects appear to be dose related. Because of the dearth of literature in this area, recommendations are that the hypnotics and sedatives only be used in the short term and that there be ongoing monitoring of the medication.

Miscellaneous Medications

This section describes a heterogeneous group of drugs that physicians may employ from time to time to manage childhood psychiatric disorders. In some cases, the evidence supporting their effectiveness is very limited. However, information about the drugs is included because school staff may encounter children who are being treated with these medications. More comprehensive information about these and other medications sometimes employed to manage childhood and adolescent mental disorders can be found in standard pharmacology and psychopharmacology texts (Green, 1995; Hardman et al., 1996; Rosenberg et al., 1994; Werry & Aman, 1993b).

Clonidine

Approximately 30% of children with ADHD do not improve with stimulant medication (R. T. Brown et al., in press). In light of this, clinicians often seek alternative medications for children suffering from this disorder. Clonidine is an antihypertensive drug that reduces the symptoms of ADHD (Hunt, Minderaa, & Cohen, 1985). It may be useful for the management of children with ADHD when the stimulants and tricyclic medications are ineffective or when adverse side effects experienced with these medications preclude their use.

Pharmacology and Pharmacokinetics. Peak plasma levels of clonidine occur between 3 and 5 hours after ingestion. The medication is a selective alpha$_2$-adrenergic agonist that acts to inhibit the release of norepinephrine. The majority of the medication is excreted unchanged by the kidneys while a lesser amount is metabolized by the liver.

Clinical Effects. The major use of clonidine is to treat hypertension. However, in a double-blind placebo-controlled crossover trial with 10 children ages 8–13 years with ADHD, Hunt et al. (1985) reported that clonidine improved hyperactivity, impulsivity, and inattention. Furthermore, they suggested that clonidine appeared to facilitate more goal-directed behavior and less oppositional behavior. Subsequent reports by this research group (Hunt, Capper, & O'Connell, 1990) suggested that children can be maintained on clonidine without loss of its effectiveness. These reports encourage the use of clonidine as an alternative to stimulants and tricyclic medications for the management of ADHD.

Adverse Side Effects and Toxicity. A major adverse side effect of clonidine is sedation which can interfere with children's work at school. In addition, children may experience hypotension and depressive symptoms (Green, 1995). As a result, clonidine should be avoided with children and adolescents who have a history of depressive symptoms or a history of cardiovascular disease. The medication also should not be used if a child has a history of an allergic reaction to clonidine or major renal disease. Overdosage with clonidine may lead to cardiac arrhythmias and seizures, so any overdose should be treated as a medical emergency.

Dosage and Administration. An interesting feature of clonidine is the possibility of using skin patches to deliver the medication (Rosenberg et al., 1994). In general, however, children experiencing mental disorders take the drug orally. To avoid some of the adverse side effects of sedation, children can take clonidine late in the evening before they go to bed.

Clonidine must be withdrawn gradually to avoid the possibility of rebound hypertension. It is important that parents and children be advised of this effect and that children do not abruptly discontinue their medication.

Summary. Clonidine is an antihypertensive medication with some potential to manage symptoms associated with ADHD, particularly when stimulants are ineffective or associated with too many adverse side effects. Adverse side effects of clonidine include hypotension and depressive symptoms, so clonidine should be avoided if patients have a history of these diseases.

Propranolol

Propranolol is the prototype of a group of medications known as beta-adrenergic blockers. Propranolol blocks the actions of epinephrine and norepinephrine. It is primarily used for treating cardiovascular disorders such as hypertension, but it is also employed to manage a range of psychiatric disorders, particularly anxiety disorders, in adults.

Pharmacology and Pharmacokinetics. Propranolol is rapidly absorbed after oral administration, but a substantial proportion of the medication is then rapidly metabolized by the liver. As a result, blood levels vary considerably after oral administration (Hardman et al., 1996).

Clinical Effects. Propranolol is used primarily to treat cardiovascular disorders. However, a direct effect of the medication's action on the autonomic nervous system is a reduction in many of the somatic symptoms of anxiety such as palpitations, sweating, and tremulousness. This effect has encouraged research investigating the effectiveness of propranolol to manage anxiety disorders in adults. In children, the medication is also used to manage aggressive disorders (Werry & Aman, 1993b). Few studies investigated the effectiveness of this medication for treating children and adolescents.

Adverse Side Effects and Toxicity. A number of adverse side effects can arise from the use of propranolol with children (e.g., diabetes, cardiovascular disorders, and respiratory disorders such as asthma). Propranolol also interacts negatively with a range of other psychotropic medications including phenothiazines, clonidine, and MAOIs. As with many of the medications described in this section, overdosage with propranolol should be treated as a medical emergency.

Dosage and Administration. There are no clear guidelines for dosage levels of propranolol for pediatric populations with psychiatric disorders. It is important to assess carefully a child's physical status before initiating the drug and to monitor the child carefully during the course of medication.

Summary. Propranolol, an antihypertensive, is employed with adults for the management of anxiety disorders. There are few trials to guide the clinical use of propranolol with children. Coupled with its side-effect profile, this warrants judicious use and scrupulous monitoring of the drug when used with this population.

CONCLUSIONS

A number of psychotropic agents are available to manage psychiatric disorders in children and adolescents. However, most of these agents were originally designed for use with adults. Often their efficacy and safety for pediatric populations remains to be researched adequately and demonstrated empirically. The psychopharmacological treatment of children involves unique developmental issues that influence both physiological and psychological factors and outcome. Issues pertaining to adherence to medication and coordination with other treatment programs are especially relevant.

Several classes of psychotropic medications tend to be used with pediatric populations. These include the stimulants, antipsychotic medications, antidepressants, lithium, antiepileptic medications, and hypnotics and sedatives. Clonidine and propranolol also are used as psychotropic agents, although their original use was in the treatment of cardiovascular disorders and hypertension.

The stimulants are the most widely used psychotropic agents for children and adolescents and the most meticulously studied. The efficacy of the stimulants is clearly documented in the management of symptoms associated with ADHD. Their side-effect profile is dose related and was found to be minimal compared with other classes of psychotropics. Both adverse and beneficial effects typically dissipate when the medication is discontinued.

The antipsychotics generally are found to be effective in reducing the symptoms associated with psychosis in children and adolescents. Although they are frequently employed to manage children and adolescents who exhibit explosiveness and aggression, the potential adverse side effects of these agents often outweigh their benefits. A major concern with these medications is the adverse neurological effects associated with long-term administration.

There is little evidence that tricyclic medications, originally developed to treat depressive disorders in adults, are effective for the treatment of depressive disorders in children and adolescents. Some recent evidence supports the efficacy of the tricyclics in managing symptoms associated with ADHD, particularly for children who have not responded satisfactorily to stimulants. The SSRIs offer advantages over the tricyclics because of their relatively safe side-effect profile. However, their clinical efficacy with children and adolescents remains to be demonstrated. The MAOIs have minimal use with pediatric populations because of their potential toxicity. They are recommended only when other medications fail and then only in very controlled inpatient settings. An emerging literature addresses the use of lithium in children and adolescents, particularly for aggression. However, until additional research is forthcoming, caution is warranted in prescribing lithium, and it must be carefully monitored for beneficial and adverse effects.

The anticonvulsants are sometimes used when children have failed other trials of psychotropic drugs. However, few empirical studies are available to guide their clinical use, and because of the cognitive toxicities associated with long-term use, judicious application and careful monitoring are necessary.

Finally, the hypnotics and sedatives have received little empirical support for managing anxiety disorders in children. Although the use of these agents in adult populations is widespread because of their relatively low side-effect profile, empirical support is far too limited to justify the regular use of these agents for children and adolescents.

CHAPTER 6

◆◆◆

Assessment and Monitoring
of Children Receiving
Psychotropic Medications

◆

This chapter describes the general approaches that psychologists can use to monitor the beneficial and adverse effects of psychotropic medication. The latter part of the chapter also provides examples of specific measures used to monitor the beneficial and adverse effects of psychotropic medications. The chapter does not attempt a comprehensive review of all the individual rating scales and observational techniques that are available to monitor child and adolescent developmental and psychiatric disorders. Several reviews already provide that information (Aman, 1993; Barkley, 1988; National Institute of Mental Health, 1985; Sattler, 1986). This chapter provides an overview of rating scales and behavioral observations that are useful for helping to determine whether a child should receive psychotropic medication as well as to monitor behaviors in response to medication.

Streiner and Norman (1995) note that the time-honored approach of asking people about how they benefited from treatment does not accurately evaluate the degree of change they experienced because "people simply do not remember how they were at the beginning" (p. 165). As a result, other approaches are needed that accurately monitor the effectiveness of treatment. Barkley, Conners, et al. (1990) pointed out that the "mandatory participation of children in public education creates a second social institution besides the family through which treatment is often administered to a child" (p. 9). This "second social institution" offers many potential advantages to monitor the effectiveness of psychotropic drugs prescribed for children and adolescents. For example, school classrooms offer many opportunities to observe behaviors such as motor movement, off-task behavior, disturbing others, and noncompliance. Interactions with peers, physical aggression, and other inappropriate social behaviors can be observed in the playground setting (Gadow & Nolan, 1993). Not only can observers view individual children in these settings, but they can also compare a child's functioning with that of peers of the same age and sex. The school setting thus offers a unique opportunity to evaluate the effectiveness of medications with children and to monitor changes in their symptoms over time.

Careful monitoring of the effects of psychotropic drugs employed to treat children and adolescents with psychiatric and developmental disorders is important for several reasons. First, the vast majority of research on the effectiveness of psychotropic drugs for the treatment of mental disorders focuses on adults. However, the effects of psychotropic drugs on children and adolescents often differ from those reported for adults (Barkley, Conners, et al., 1990; E. Taylor, 1994), including the effect of psychotropic drugs on the body (pharmacodynamics) and the effect of bodily systems on psychotropic drugs (pharmacokinetics). These differences reflect children's more rapid rate of absorption and metabolization of many drugs and the greater speed with which drugs pass through the blood–brain barrier in children (Werry & Aman, 1993b). Differences also are evident in the effect of drugs on childhood mental disorders. For example, psychotropic drugs appear less effective in treating childhood depressive disorders than in treating adult depressive disorders. These child–adult differences, along with a lack of research focusing specifically on children and adolescents, mean that physicians have to weigh carefully the possible deleterious impact of psychiatric disorders on children and adolescents against the possibility that children may receive little benefit from a psychotropic medication or may experience significant adverse effects from the medication.

Second, generally there is not a specific psychotropic drug treatment for specific illnesses, and few indicators accurately predict children's responses to specific drugs or dosages (E. Taylor, 1994). As a result, when psychotropic drugs are prescribed for children, clinicians must carefully monitor children's responses to the different drugs and different dosage levels in identifying the most effective treatment for individual children.

Third, children's social behavior and psychological and cognitive functioning are all constantly changing as the children develop. That makes monitoring of drug effects more complex. Furthermore, some medications primarily have adverse effects on the physical development of children, whereas other drugs may impede their cognitive development.

Fourth, young children are less able to report the presence of adverse effects than are adults. Thus, parents and teachers must carefully monitor the children for signs of adverse effects. This monitoring may need to extend over long periods, particularly for children who are treated with psychotropic drugs that can give rise to severe adverse effects such as tardive dyskinesia.

Fifth, children rarely initiate their own referral to physicians, and, particularly for younger children, the decision to use psychotropic drugs is based largely on information provided by parents or teachers. Indeed, young children may have little influence on decisions about whether or not they receive psychotropic drugs. This situation contrasts with that of adults who generally arrange their own referrals and who may actively seek medication to relieve their distress. The more limited influence that children have in determining their treatment places a greater responsibility on physicians, parents, and teachers to ensure that children are not exposed to adverse effects of psychotropic drugs or disadvantaged in other ways by their treatment.

Unfortunately, monitoring of beneficial and adverse effects of psychotropic medication for children and adolescents with psychiatric and developmental disorders tends to be somewhat haphazard (Gadow, Nolan, Paolicelli, & Sprafkin, 1991). Gadow et al. have drawn attention to the fact that dosage adjustments, contacts between physicians and classroom teachers, and the use of well-validated instruments often occur sporadically. Teachers often are uncertain about the medications being used by children, whereas physicians generally have limited knowledge about a child's behavior at school. Physicians tend to rely on reports from parents or caretakers, who have little opportunity to observe a child's behavior at school. As a result, they may be unaware of the adverse effects of medication on the child's cognitive functioning or the beneficial effects on the child's peer relationships.

Several approaches are available to monitor children's behavior more systematically, including behavior rating scales, direct observation, and specific devices to rate performance, academic progress, and activity. In the past, monitoring focused largely on target symptoms and potential adverse effects of psychotropic drugs. In addition, most research on monitoring focused on the effects of stimulant drugs used to treat children with ADHD. Less attention was given to the monitoring of other disorders and treatments. It is important that the monitoring of treatment effectiveness embrace a range of issues that include compliance with treatment; indirect indicators of outcome (e.g., academic progress, number of school days missed, and number of school suspensions); physical development; biochemical status, including blood tests, liver function tests, or tests for psychotropic drug levels (e.g., lithium levels); and health-related quality of life.

MONITORING PHYSICAL EFFECTS

Clinicians must take a baseline medical history and physical assessment before prescribing psychotropic medication for children (Zametkin & Yamada, 1993). This helps to rule out several other illnesses that may mimic psychiatric disorders (e.g., diseases of the CNS; various vascular disorders, infections; metabolic disorders; nutritional deficiencies; and the use or abuse of drugs, medications, or other toxic substances).

Zametkin and Yamada (1993) also recommend taking a detailed medical history, including information about immunizations, previous hospitalizations, trauma, transfusions, allergies, current medications, substance use history, social history, family medical history, and family psychiatric history. Each of these areas is important as the information may suggest poor compliance with previous health care, accident proneness, a history of abuse or neglect, such sexually transmitted diseases as human immunodeficiency virus (HIV), acquired immune deficiency syndrome (AIDS), and interactions with other drugs that are employed to treat nonpsychiatric, organic disorders. For example, a child with a history of appetite disturbances may not fare particularly well on stimulant medication because this class of drugs is demonstrated to suppress appetite. In addition, children who are particularly anxious may have a high baseline of physical or somatic complaints that could erroneously be attributed to psychotropic medication.

It is also recommended that physicians carefully review all organ systems to establish a baseline for later assessment of adverse side effects of various medications. As Zametkin and Yamada (1993) pointed out, psychotropic drugs affect many organ systems. For example, stimulants, antidepressants, and neuroleptic agents all have significant effects on the cardiovascular systems, including heart rate and blood pressure. Psychotropic agents may interact with other pharmacological therapies used to manage other childhood disorders, such as asthma, and also may interact physiologically with other organ systems, such as the cardiovascular system. The review of organ systems should include the eyes, ears, nose, and throat; the respiratory, cardiovascular, gastrointestinal, urinary, genital, and reproductive tracts; and musculoskeletal, skin, endocrine, and central nervous systems.

Before initiating a trial of any psychotropic medication, clinicians should undertake a psychiatric review of the child or adolescent to identify any symptoms related to psychosis, including hallucinations and delusions and obsessions and compulsions. Because some psychiatric symptoms reflect adverse side effects of psychotropic medications, it is important for clinicians to evaluate such symptoms during the course of medication treatment.

A physical and neurological examination also provides a baseline against which to evaluate adverse physical effects of psychotropic medication, (e.g., on blood pressure, pulse rate, and height and weight). The clinician should carefully evaluate the patient for tics, particularly children receiving stimulant medication (Zametkin & Yamada, 1993). The physical examination can include tests for specific diagnoses (e.g., thyroid studies to evaluate for depression) and to determine whether prescribed psychotropic medication is affecting organ systems (e.g., liver function tests for children treated with pemoline.

Finally, many psychotropic agents, including the stimulants, neuroleptics, and tricyclic antidepressants, have the potential to alter speech and language abilities, including speech production, rate, volume, and coherence. For this reason, researchers recommend that, as a screen for age-appropriate language skills, the clinician conduct a baseline assessment, informally interacting with the child and noting any abnormalities in articulation.

ASSESSMENT OF ADVERSE PHYSICAL EFFECTS

Because children and adolescents frequently do not complain overtly about physical problems and, at times, find it difficult to describe physical symptoms, it is imperative to monitor adverse physical side effects in a systematic manner (Zametkin & Yamada, 1993). Children's potentially greater sensitivity to pharmacotherapy also makes systematic and ongoing monitoring of adverse side effects crucial. Parents are important as informants about any adverse side effects associated with their children's pharmacotherapy.

Several approaches are available for systematic assessment of adverse medication effects in children and adolescents. These include rating scales, checklists, physical and neurological examinations, laboratory studies, and electrophysiological (EEG or EKG) studies. Rating scales have an advantage in assessing adverse side effects of pharmacotherapy in that these measures may elicit symptoms that a parent or child may not spontaneously report. Several excellent rating scales are available for the assessment of physical side effects, including the Dosage Record and Treatment Emergent Symptom Scale (DOTES; Guy, 1976a), the Subjective Treatment Emergent Symptom Scale (STESS; Guy, 1976b), the Abnormal Involuntary Movement Scale (AIMS; Guy, 1976c), and the NIMH Systematic Assessment for Treatment Emergent Events (SAFTEE-GI; M. Campbell & Palij, 1985). These rating scales assess physical and CNS effects and are appropriate for use with both adults and children (Zametkin & Yamada, 1993). An exhaustive review of all the available rating scales for adverse physical effects is not possible within the scope of this chapter, but readers are encouraged to examine M. Campbell and Palij (1985) and

M. Campbell, Green, and Deutsch (1985). However, Zametkin and Yamada (1993) caution that although rating scales offer a systematic means
of assessing adverse side effects, the development of these scales is often
based on studies with adult populations. Thus, they recommend that
checklists be used with care by physicians in a way that is appropriate for
pediatric populations. Appendix A presents a rating scale, developed by
Barkley et al. (1993), for children that assesses adverse side effects associated with stimulants.

Researchers also recommend that neurological examinations be a
routine part of monitoring for adverse side effects in children and adolescents. Over the years, there were efforts to quantify the CNS response of
various psychotropics, and several assessment batteries are available for
use by practitioners, including the Physical and Neurological Examination
of Soft Signs (PANESS; Guy, 1976d), which was revised in recent years.
Numerous methodological difficulties and psychometric problems characterize neurological assessments, and future research efforts need to focus
on developing a standardized neurological examination to quantify many
of the adverse neurological effects associated with some psychotropics. It
should be noted, however, that the "soft signs" component of the neurological examination is no longer considered useful in the monitoring of
drug effects (R. T. Brown et al., in press).

Laboratory measures of physical functioning include the EKG to
identify cardiac arrhythmias associated with tricyclic antidepressants.
Other laboratory screening tests may include thyroid function tests, catecholamine and enzyme assays, screening for HIV, EEG, and routine liver,
kidney, and serum measures. These laboratory tests also may prove useful
in evaluating the etiology of psychiatric symptoms or monitoring drug effects on organ functioning (Zametkin & Yamada, 1993). The dexamethasone suppression test was previously believed to be associated with major
depression, but its validity has been questioned in recent years (Klee &
Garfinkel, 1984; Zametkin & Yamada, 1993).

Literature is emerging that pertains to genetic studies and brain
imaging in children and adolescents (Brown & Donegan, 1995). For example, significant progress has been made in identifying genetic markers for
specific psychiatric and developmental disorders in pediatric populations
(Zametkin & Yamada, 1993), and behavioral genetics is an area ripe for
future study. Similarly, researchers extensively studied the use of radiographic tests of brain imaging, including computerized tomography
(CT), magnetic resonance imaging (MRI), EEG spectral tomography, and
PET, for children with various developmental and psychiatric disorders
(R. T. Brown & Donegan, 1995). However, the routine use of these tests to
predict or monitor drug response is not common, and their high costs
make it unlikely that they will ever be used routinely.

ASSESSMENT OF BEHAVIOR, EMOTION, AND COGNITION

Assessment instruments help quantify frequency and severity of symptoms and evaluate the efficacy of a particular therapy. Instruments frequently employed to monitor drug efficacy often have been found to be sensitive to the effects of various pharmacotherapies. Just as objective and psychometrically valid assessments must be employed to diagnose specific psychiatric and developmental disorders, assessments also are necessary to evaluate the effects of psychotropic drug therapy. Typically, assessments of medication response include structured interviews, rating scales, direct observations of behavior, and measures of performance, achievement, and activity.

Structured Interviews

Aman (1993) described four types of interview format to diagnose psychiatric disorders and assess the effectiveness of either psychotherapy or pharmacotherapy. These include unstructured, semistructured, and structured interviews, and symptom checklists. The unstructured interview is the most common format in clinical practice, but with the advent of greater precision in diagnostic practice fostered by DSM-IV (American Psychiatric Association, 1994), structured interviews have become more readily available in recent years. However, structured interviews present a practical problem in administration for the assessment of drug efficacy because of their length and their questionable sensitivity and specificity in identifying individual symptoms of disorders. The semistructured interview offers some compromise between structured and unstructured interviews, although it requires significant training on the part of the interviewer. Reliable semistructured interview instruments include the Diagnostic Interview for Children (DICA; Herjanic & Reich, 1982) and the Kiddie–Schedule for Affective Disorders and Schizophrenia (K-SADS; Chambers et al., 1985). Symptom checklists provide practitioners with prompts to make certain they cover all major areas of a psychiatric diagnosis. Recently, computer algorithms have become available to enhance reliability.

Behavior Rating Scales

Behavior rating scales have several advantages. They are economical and normative data may be available for comparisons with the ratings of individual children. Relevant behaviors can be sampled across different settings and across time, and data can be gathered on rare or infrequent behaviors. Finally, substantial information is available about the psychometric properties of many scales (Conners & Barkley, 1985). Well-constructed rating scales also are sensitive to the effects of various psychotropic drugs (M. Campbell et al., 1985).

However, rating scales have limitations, including the possibility that results are influenced by characteristics of the person completing the rating scale. Further, it may be difficult to establish a baseline score because a second rating often shows a score reduction that does not seem to reflect improvements in children's behavior. For this reason, investigators suggest that baseline assessments include two ratings of children's behavior. Finally, children with problems in one area may be incorrectly reported as having problems in several other areas. Broadly based behavior scales often do not provide adequate ratings of children with low incidence or very severe psychiatric disorders such as childhood schizophrenia or autism. Table 6.1 presents the most widely employed rating scales for evaluating the effects of psychotropic medications in children.

As can be seen in Table 6.1, many rating scales are available to monitor medication effects in children and adolescents. These include general scales, preschool rating scales, and rating scales that assess specific disorders such as ADHD and other disruptive behavioral disorders (e.g., oppositional defiant disorder, conduct disorders, and aggression; depression, mood disorders, manic–depressive disorders, and mania; anxiety disorders; schizophrenia; tic and Tourette's disorders; mental retardation; and autism) (Aman, 1993). This chapter briefly addresses the primary rating scales employed for each major disorder.

Measurement of Emotional, Behavioral, and Social Competencies

Because of time limitations, practitioners are often limited to only one measure in their assessment battery. For this reason, most outpatient clinics employ general rating scales that are appropriate for assessing children and adolescents.

The Child Behavior Checklist (CBCL) is employed most frequently as a general index of psychopathology (Achenbach, 1991a). Emotional and behavioral problems and social competence can be assessed by means of the CBCL completed by parents, the Teacher Report Form (TRF) completed by teachers, and the Youth Self-Report (YSR) completed by adolescents (Achenbach, 1991a, 1991b, 1991c). These self-administered checklists provide comparable information from parents and teachers, and extensive data support their reliability and validity. The checklists consist of two parts. The first part obtains information about social competencies, and the second part assesses a wide range of behavior problems. Eight

TABLE 6.1. Summary of Rating Scales

Rating scale	Target problem or population	Rater					Psychometric characteristics
		Clinician	Parent	Child	Teacher		

Rating scale	Target problem or population	Clinician	Parent	Child	Teacher	Psychometric characteristics
Aberrant Behavior Checklist (plus others, contingent upon specific behavior problems)	Mental retardation, autism		✓	✓	✓	Good test–retest reliability; adequate interrater reliability; good criterion group validity
ADD-H Adolescent Self-Report Scale	ADHD			✓		Unavailable
ADHD Comprehensive Teacher Rating Scale	ADHD				✓	Good interrater reliability; sensitive to stimulant medication
ADHD Rating Scale	ADHD		✓		✓	Excellent internal consistency; good test–retest reliability, and validity
Anxiety Disorders Interview Schedule	Anxiety		✓	✓		Satisfactory test–retest reliability
Attention Checklist	Mental retardation				✓	Sensitivity to pharmacological treatments largely untested
Preschool Behavior Checklist	Preschool children		✓			Psychometrics established
Behavior Problems Inventory (aggression and self-injury	Mental retardation		✓		✓	Variable reliability ranging from poor to excellent

(continued)

133

TABLE 6.1. (*continued*)

Rating scale	Target problem or population	Rater				Psychometric characteristics
		Clinician	Parent	Child	Teacher	
Behavioral Screening Questionnaire	Preschool children				✓	Convergent validity with clinical assessment
Bellevue Index of Depression	Depressive disorders	✓	✓		✓	High validity
Child Anxiety Frequency Checklist	Anxiety			✓		Moderate test–retest reliability; moderate to high internal consistency
Child Behavior Checklist/2–3	Ages 2–3 years		✓			Acceptable to good psychometrics
Child Behavior Checklist	General purpose, 4 years and older		✓			High test–retest reliability; good content validity and criterion validity
Child Depression Scale	Depressive disorders			✓		High internal consistency and convergent validity; poor correspondence with parent and teacher ratings
Childhood Anxiety Frequency Checklist	Anxiety			✓		Moderate reliability and internal consistency
Childhood Anxiety Sensitivity Index	Anxiety			✓		Moderate to high test–retest reliability; moderate internal consistency
Childhood Attention Problems Scale	ADHD				✓	Adequate reliability and validity; drug sensitive

Instrument	Disorder/Use				Comments
Children's Depression Inventory (parent and teacher versions)	Depressive disorders	✓			Variable agreement between parent and teacher ratings
Children's Depression Inventory	Depressive disorders		✓		High test–retest reliability and validity; low specificity
Children's Depression Rating Scale—Revised	Depressive disorders			✓	Acceptable internal consistency; test–retest reliability, and parent–child agreement
Children's Depression Scale	Depressive disorders (parent and teacher version)	✓			Moderate agreement with child ratings
Children's Inventory of Anger	Oppositional defiant disorder, conduct disorder; aggression		✓		Psychometric data unknown; drug sensitive
Children's Psychiatric Rating Scale	Autism			✓	High interrater reliability; validity unstudied; sensitive to psychotropic medication
Clinical Global Impressions	General purpose			✓	Psychometrics largely unknown and vary across clinical populations
Conners Abbreviated Symptom Questionnaire	ADHD, autism	✓			Assesses hyperactivity and emotional lability; drug sensitive
Conners Teacher Rating Scale	Oppositional defiant conduct, aggression	✓			High test–retest reliability and validity; variable interrater reliability; some subscales drug sensitive
Conners Parent Rating Scale	ADHD, oppositional defiant disorder; conduct disorder; aggression	✓			Drug sensitive (longer version)

(continued)

135

TABLE 6.1. (continued)

Rating scale	Target problem or population	Rater				Psychometric characteristics
		Clinician	Parent	Child	Teacher	
Depressive Self-Rating Scale	Depressive disorders			✓		
Developmentally Delayed Children's Behavior Checklist	Mental retardation, autism		✓		✓	Sensitivity to pharmacological treatment largely untested
Devereux Adolescent Behavior Rating Scale	Mental retardation		✓		✓	
Devereux Child Behavior Rating Scale	Mental retardation		✓		✓	
Diagnostic Interview for Depression in Children and Adolescents	Depressive disorders	✓				High reliability and validity
DSM-Derived Scales	Anxiety	✓	✓	✓	✓	
Emotional Disorders Rating Scale	Depressive disorders, anxiety		✓		✓	Low test–retest reliability; high interrater reliability
Emotional Disorders Rating Scale for Developmental Disabilities	Mental retardation		✓		✓	No data on treatment sensitivity
Fear Survey Schedule for Children	Anxiety			✓		High internal consistency; good test–retest reliability
Home Situations Questionnaire	ADHD		✓			Moderately high test–retest reliability; unkown interrater reliability; sensitive to stimulant medication

Instrument	Disorder/Focus	Comments
Interview Schedule for Children	Depressive disorders	Structured interview
Iowa Conners Teacher's Rating Scale	Oppositional defiant disorder, conduct disorder, aggression, hyperactivity	High test–retest reliability and internal consistency; drug sensitive
Leyton Obsessional Inventory—Child	Obsessive–compulsive disorder	Good test–retest reliability; only moderate specificity for obsessive–compulsive disorder
Louisville Behavior Checklist	Anxiety	Discriminant validity; high split-half reliabilities
Louisville Fear Survey for Children	Anxiety	Discriminant validity; high split-half reliabilities
Maladaptive Behavior Scale	General purpose	Primarily for residential-type settings
Manic-State Rating Scale	Bipolar disorder	Reliable; valid; difficult to administer
Overt Aggression Scale	Oppositional defiant disorder, conduct disorder, aggression	Psychometric studies largely from adults; used in inpatient settings with severely aggressive patients; drug sensitivity largely unknown
Peer Conflict Scale	Oppositional defiant disorder, conduct disorder, aggression	High associations with direct observation of noncompliance; high test–retest reliability; some evidence of drug sensitivity

(continued)

TABLE 6.1. (*continued*)

| Rating scale | Target problem or population | Rater | | | | | Psychometric characteristics |
		Clinician	Parent	Child	Teacher		
Peer Nomination Inventory of Depression	Depressive disorders			✓		Peer ratings	
Preschool Behavior Questionnaire	Preschool children		✓		✓	Adequate interrater and-test–retest reliability; high discrimination between community and clinic children	
Rating Scale of Dysphoria	Depressive disorders		✓		✓	Not psychometrically robust; poor content validity	
Real Life Rating Scale	Autism	✓				Unknown test–retest reliability; some studies show drug sensitivity	
Revised Behavior Problem Checklist	General purpose		✓		✓	Adequate interrater reliability; internal consistency high; good criterion validity	
Revised Children's Manifest Anxiety Scale	Anxiety			✓		Good specificity; low sensitivity; drug sensitivity not high	
Reynolds Adolescent Depression Scale	Depressive disorders			✓		High internal consistency, test–retest reliability, and convergent validity	
Schedule for Affective Disorders and Schizphrenia for School-Age Children	Depressive disorders	✓				Adequate reliability and validity	

138

Instrument	Disorder/Population			Comments
Schedule for Affective Disorders and Schizophrenia for School-Age Children (modified for repeated ratings)	Anxiety	✓		Excellent test–retest reliability; concurrent validity supported
School-Age Depression Listed Inventory	Depressive disorders	✓		Structured interview
School Situations Questionnaire	ADHD	✓	✓	Moderately high test–retest reliability; unknown interrater reliability; sensitive to stimulant medication
Self-Injurious Behavior Questionnaire	Mental retardation		✓	Sensitivity to pharmacological treatments largely untested
Social Dysfunction and Aggression Scale	Oppositional defiant disorder, conduct disorder, aggression	✓		High interrater reliability
Staff Observation Aggression Scale	Oppositional defiant disorder, conduct disorder, aggression	✓		Psychometric studies largely from adults; used in inpatient settings with severely aggressive patients; drug sensitivity largely unknown
State–Trait Anxiety Inventory for Children	Anxiety		✓	Norms available only for 4th–6th grade; high test–retest reliability; good specificity; poor sensitivity
Stony Brook	Schizophrenia	✓		Psychometrically promising; no evidence of drug response
Symptom Checklist	Preschool children	✓		Derived from factor analysis of behavior ratings

(continued)

TABLE 6.1. ***(continued)***

		Rater				
Rating scale	Target problem or population	Clinician	Parent	Child	Teacher	Psychometric characteristics
Teacher Report Form	General purpose				✓	Psychometrics good; drug sensitivity unknown
Timed Stereotypies Ratings Scale	Autism	✓				Drug sensitive
Tourette Syndrome Global Scale	Tic and Tourette's	✓				High reliability and drug sensitivity
Tourette Syndrome Severity Scale	Tic and Tourette's	✓				High reliability and drug sensitivity
Werry–Weiss–Peters Activity Scale	ADHD		✓			Low specificity; drug sensitive
Yale Children's Inventory	ADHD		✓			Satisfactory internal consistency, test–retest reliability, and discriminant validity
Yale Global Tic Severity Scale	Tic and Tourette's	✓				Psychometrically robust
Youth Self-Report	Oppositional defiant disorder, conduct disorder, aggression			✓		Subscales for assessing delinquent and aggressive behaviors; problems with underreporting via self-report

syndrome scales (or narrow-band factors) labeled Withdrawn, Somatic Complaints, Anxious/Depressed, Social Problems, Thought Problems, Attention Problems, Delinquent Behavior, and Aggressive Behavior are scored from this part of the checklist. In addition, there are two broadly based scales labeled Internalizing and Externalizing. The Internalizing score describes fearful, inhibited, and overcontrolled behaviors, and the Externalizing score rates aggressive, antisocial, and undercontrolled behavior. A total behavior problem score comprising all the behavior items on the checklist is also scored. The relatively long period over which the checklists assess behavior limits their value in assessing pharmacotherapy.

A brief and useful measure (the Childhood Attention Problems Scale; Edelbrock, 1978) that was derived from the TRF has good reliability and validity and is frequently employed to assess stimulant drug response (see Appendix B). This measure extracts items that have loaded on the Hyperactivity narrow band factor and that were consistent with DSM-III-R (American Psychological Association, 1987) criteria for ADHD.

Measurement of Attention-Deficit/Hyperactivity Disorder

A number of parent, teacher, and child rating scales are available to assess symptoms associated with ADHD. To date, self-ratings have not been entirely successful when employed alone in the identification of children with externalizing disorders, primarily because of children's and adolescents' underreporting of symptoms. Also, their use in assessing children's perceptions of symptom changes from pharmacotherapy is not entirely clear and will be an important focus of future research. A widely used set of rating scales are the Conners Rating Scales.

There are five versions of the Conners Parent and Teacher Rating Scales, two for parents and three for teachers (Conners, 1970; Conners & Barkley, 1985; Goyette, Conners, & Ulrich, 1978). The major difference between the two versions of the parent questionnaire is the number of items in each version. The original parent questionnaire consisted of 93 items; the subsequent version reduced the number to 48 items and reworded some items to simplify administration and interpretation. Conners and Barkley (1985) noted that the parent scale shows a consistent practice effect between the first and second administration, with scores generally being lower at the second administration. As a result, they suggest that it is desirable to have at least two baseline assessments before any trial of medication.

There are three versions of the teacher rating scales, containing 39 items, 28 items, and 10 items, respectively (Conners, 1969; Conners & Barkley, 1985; Goyette et al., 1978). Conners and Barkley (1985) noted some confusion about the 10-item scale because of variations in the item content and the method of scoring reported in some publications. They advise using the version of the questionnaire described in the article by Goyette et al. (1978). They explain that the scale described in the article shows "a high degree of sensitivity to drug effects, particularly with the stimulants, and is most appropriate when many repeated measures are required from either parents or teachers" (Conners & Barkley, 1985, p. 810).

Measurement of Childhood Depressive Disorders

There have been few controlled clinical trials of antidepressant medication with children and adolescents, and, for this reason, the validity of depression rating scales in assessment of drug efficacy is uncertain (Aman, 1993). Recommendations are that several sources (e.g., teachers, parents, and children) be involved in the assessment of treatment response. The value of depression rating scales in drug trials is complicated by the fact that changes in depression ratings may occur independent of treatment efficacy because ratings tend to improve with repeated administration.

The Children's Depression Inventory (CDI) is a 27-item self-report scale designed to identify a range of depressive symptoms (Kovacs, 1985). Each item includes three statements that reflect increasing severity of depressive symptoms. Children or adolescents completing the scale choose the statement that best describes their feelings or ideas over the past 2 weeks. Although the CDI is widely used to assess childhood depression, it is unclear how sensitive it is to detect changes in children's depressive symptoms during drug trials.

Measurement of Childhood Anxiety Disorders

Few well-controlled psychotropic drug trials have been conducted with anxiety disorders in children (Aman, 1993). For this reason, there are few guidelines to help practitioners identify which rating scales are actually sensitive to drug effects. Klein (1988) recommended that any assessment of drug effects include an evaluation of both state and trait anxiety. State anxiety is regarded as transitory and is a response to a particular stressor, whereas trait anxiety is deemed to reflect a stable characteristic of the child's personality (Aman, 1993).

Revised Children's Manifest Anxiety Scale. The Revised Children's Manifest Anxiety Scale is widely used to quantify anxiety symptoms experienced by children and adolescents (Reynolds & Paget, 1983). The scale consists of 37 statements to which children respond with "yes" or "no," depending on whether they believe the statement is true about themselves. Again, although the scale was used in a large number of studies of childhood anxiety, there is limited information about its capacity to detect changes in drug trials.

The Leyton Obsessional Inventory—Child Version. Obsessive–compulsive disorder is a specific anxiety disorder experienced by adults and children. It is characterized by repetitive intrusive thoughts and rituals that are both chronic and distressing to the patient. The Leyton Obsessional Inventory, an assessment tool for adults, was modified to make it suitable for use with children and adolescents (C. J. Berg, Rapoport, & Flament, 1986). There are two versions of the instrument, one consisting of 20 items, which is intended for use in surveys, and the other consisting of 44 items, which is designed for the assessment of children and adolescents with obsessive-compulsive disorder. The items ask about a range of symptoms of obsessive-compulsive disorder, and the 44-item version is reported to have excellent test–retest reliability and to be sensitive to the effects of psychotropic medications.

Measurement of Health-Related Quality of Life

Treatment outcome studies increasingly incorporate ratings of consumer satisfaction, quality of life, and the general health status of children. The Child Health Questionnaire is a recently developed measure of children's health status and it includes a parent and a child version (Landgraf, Abetz, & Ware, 1997). The child version consists of 87 items, and there are two versions of the parent questionnaire, one containing 50 items and the other containing 28 items. Both the parent-completed and child-completed versions evaluate children's functioning in a range of areas, including physical, social, and family functioning.

Direct Observations of Behavior

Direct observation is best employed to assess high-frequency behavior and global behaviors (Sattler, 1986). Sattler identified a number of advantages of the direct observation method. Specifically, direct observation provides a cohesive picture of children's spontaneous behavior in everyday settings, such as the classroom, playground, home, or hospital ward, and in special settings such as a clinic or playroom. Thus, a distinct advantage of direct observation is its high ecological validity. Further, direct observation provides information about children's interpersonal behavior and learning styles. In addition, direct observation provides a systematic record of both children's behavior and the behaviors of others that can be used for evaluation and intervention planning.

Another advantage of direct observation is that it helps verify the accuracy of parent and teacher reports about the child's behavior. Direct observation also allows for comparisons between behaviors in test situations and those occurring in more naturalistic settings. Behavioral observations are especially useful in studying young children and children who are developmentally disabled and who may not be easily evaluated by other procedures. Direct observations can be repeated frequently without practice effects and can be used with disturbed or uncooperative children. Finally, direct observation can be tailored to focus on the specific problems of individual children.

Limitations of direct observation include its expense and the logistical difficulty in arranging it. Further, the sampling period over which behavior is observed may not be representative of children's behavior at other points of time or in other settings. Direct observation also focuses largely on observable behavior rather than on children's internal distress. Finally, observer drift may lead to changes in the ratings of children that reflect observer fatigue or forgetfulness rather than changes in children's behavior. Observer drift is particularly important if observations are extended over long periods. These issues make it important to ensure that the behaviors to be observed are clearly defined and that observation times and settings are chosen with care.

In support of direct observational methodologies, DuPaul and Kyle (1995) noted that not only can changes within a specific behavioral domain vary across dosages, but that different behaviors may be affected differentially by medication at the same dose. For example, with stimulant medication for children diagnosed with ADHD, it was demonstrated that cognition is best enhanced with a lower dose of medication, whereas behavior improved with a relatively higher dose of the same medication (R. T. Brown & Sleator, 1979; Sprague & Sleator, 1977). Moreover, some investigators have provided convincing evidence that children may vary idiosyncratically in their behavior as a function of the dose of a medication (Rapport, et al., 1986). For this reason, DuPaul and Kyle (1995) recommend that behavior change be evaluated across doses on an individual basis by means of single-subject design methodologies.

Several types of direct observational methods are available, including continuous records, response duration, frequency counts, interval recordings, and momentary time sampling. Interval recordings are typically used in psychopharmacology studies whereby several categories of behavior are monitored and specific behaviors are sampled within an interval period (e.g., 30 seconds).

A number of observational codes are available for various psychiatric and developmental disorders in children and adolescents. For example, several coding schemes are available to assess ADHD, conduct disorder, aggression, depression, and anxiety disorders (Aman, 1993). Examples of behavioral categories used to assess ADHD include off-task behaviors, noncompliance, gross motor movements, out-of-chair behaviors, fidgeting, verbalizations, and vocalizations. Examples of behavioral categories used to assess conduct disorder or aggression include physical aggression, verbal aggression, and noncompliance. Examples of behaviors to sample depression and anxiety include prosocial initiation, social isolation, inactivity, crying or whimpering, posturing, stuttering, and tremor. Two examples of direct observation codes are included below.

Attention-Deficit/Hyperactivity Disorder School Observation Code

The Attention-Deficit/Hyperactivity Disorder School Observation Code (Nolan, Gadow, & Sverd, 1994) was designed for observations of children with ADHD in classrooms, lunchrooms, and playgrounds. The measure assesses children's classroom behavior in five areas: interference, motor movement, noncompliance, nonphysical aggression, and off-task behavior. The lunchroom and playground are settings in which appropriate social behavior, noncompliance, nonphysical aggression, physical aggression, and verbal aggression can be employed in the assessments. Information is available about both the reliability and validity of the measure. Training in its use is not difficult, and teachers or school psychologists can readily use it to observe children in their natural classroom or other school settings.

Direct Observation Form

The Direct Observation Form (DOF) is suitable for recording observations of children in classrooms and other group settings (Achenbach & Edelbrock, 1983). Its authors recommend that DOF scores be averaged over a minimum of three 10-minute observations made on different occasions during the day. Like the child behavior checklists, externalizing and internalizing scores may be obtained from the results of the observations. In addition, testers can also obtain several narrow band syndrome scores.

Measures of Performance, Academic Achievement, and Activity

The development of psychological test instruments to assess drug response has been an enterprising endeavor among test publishers. However, psychological testing is merely one facet of a comprehensive test battery used to evaluate a child during a trial of medication. Psychological tests always should be used simultaneously with behavioral observations, teacher and parent ratings of behavior, and sociometric ratings. Many different types of cognitive assessments are available for the psychologist interested in assessing a child's responses to medication. These assessments include performance tests, computerized assessments, and intelligence and achievement tests (Aman, 1993).

Performance Tests

Performance tests measure cognitive functioning by assessing specific performance on a task. The child or adolescent is typically required to perform some type of action that is believed to measure a specific cognitive function. Shelton and Barkley (1995) pointed out that performance on measures of cognitive functioning is likely to be confounded by other abilities or impairments, including mental and linguistic abilities, memory, and executive functions. Recent research also indicates that laboratory measures have only moderate construct validity at best, and such instruments frequently fall short of predicting important abilities such as attentional problems. This is the case in key settings like the classroom (Barkley, 1991; Shelton & Barkley, 1995), where children with specific behavioral problems such as ADHD are likely to be encountered and to exhibit significant difficulties with behavior. Additional normative data are necessary for the majority of cognitive tests that are used in psychotropic drug trials with children (Shelton & Barkley, 1995).

Specific tests commonly used in pediatric psychopharmacology include the Continuous Performance Task (CPT) (for review, see Aman, 1978), Cancellation Tasks (for review, see Barkley, 1991), the Matching Familiar Figures Task (MFF; Kagan, 1965), the Paired Associate Learning (PAL; Swanson, 1985), the Delay Task (M. Gordon, 1983), the Short Term Recognition Memory Task (Sprague & Sleator, 1977), and the Automated Measures of Activity Level (Conners & Kronsberg, 1985). Aman (1993) has provided a comprehensive review of these tests.

The primary limitation of performance measures is their modest ecological validity. Some measures, such as the MFF, are also inconsistent in discriminating clinical groups from controls (for review, see Aman, 1993). In addition, many of these tasks, including the MFF and the Delay Task, are insensitive to stimulant medication. Shelton and Barkley (1995) reviewed recent research pertaining to CPT, a laboratory-based measure that requires the child to focus on a screen while searching for a particular stimulus. Although the ease of administration makes this assessment device intuitively appealing, its high rate of false positives and false negatives casts doubt on the validity and clinical utility of this measure in accurately identifying response to medication (DuPaul, Anastopoulos, Shelton, Guevremont, & Metevia, 1992). Similarly, another widely used instrument in drug trials of children with ADHD—the MFF—is inconsistent in its ability to discriminate children with behavioral disorders from their typically developing peers (R. T. Brown & Quay, 1977) and is of questionable specificity. The MFF has been associated with intellectual functioning (Milich & Kramer, 1985). Many of these performance tests, including the CPT, the Cancellation Tasks, and the PAL, at times appear sensitive in discriminating clinical groups (particularly those with ADHD from normally developing children) and are sensitive to stimulant medication, but other, more valid assessment techniques such as teacher and parent ratings and direct observations, should be included in the assessment battery. Under no circumstances should performance measures be the sole assessment method for assessing a child or evaluating psychotropic drug effects.

Computerized Assessment

The advent of computer technology has spawned an interest in computerized assessment of psychotropic drug effects. Aman (1993) documented the advantages and disadvantages of computerized assessments for monitoring cognitive effects of psychotropic medications. Advantages include objectivity and standardization of assessments, culture-fair assessments, precision in the recording of test responses, novelty of the tasks, the capacity of computers to handle multiple inputs, and immediate scoring and results. Disadvantages include the high cost of computer technology and software, fragility of equipment, possible loss of equivalence from the paper-and-pencil format to the computer format, questionable ecological validity, and a lack of standardization and normative data.

Two computerized vigilance tasks that are widely used to assess drug response in children with ADHD include the Gordon Diagnostic System and the Test of Variables of Attention (TOVA; Greenberg & Waldman, 1993). The Gordon Diagnostic System is criticized because it lacks sensitivity to stimulants (Aman, 1993), although some studies have demonstrated stimulant drug effects on the measure (R. T. Brown, Jaffe, Silverstein, & McGee, 1991; R. T. Brown & Sexson, 1988). Norms for the TOVA are available, and it appears to be sensitive to stimulant drug effects, although we need more data before endorsing its efficacy.

Intelligence and Achievement Tests

Tests of intelligence or mental abilities are frequently used when assessing medication effects. However, because these measures and the underlying constructs are fairly stable and are global indices of mental abilities, it is not surprising that their sensitivity to psychotropic drug effects has not been demonstrated (Aman, 1993). One exception is the Porteus Maze Test (Porteus, 1967), consisting of a set of mazes that increase in complexity as the child progresses through the task. The test assesses vigilance and attention. Although the Porteus Maze Test is sensitive to medication effects (Aman, 1993), it is only moderately associated with other measures of mental abilities.

Many children who are treated with psychotropic medication also suffer from difficulties in learning and, hence, academic achievement. As a consequence, many psychologists are involved in assessing the academic achievement of children and adolescents who are receiving psychotropic medication. Numerous achievement tests that assess psychotropic drug effects are used in drug studies with pediatric populations. These include the Wide Range Achievement Test (Jastak & Wilkinson, 1990), the Woodcock–Johnson Psychoeducational Battery—Revised (Woodcock, 1989), and the Gilmore Oral Reading Test (for review, see Gadow, 1985). As noted by Brown and associates (R. T. Brown & Borden, 1989; R. T. Brown et al., 1997, in press), it is difficult to assess the effects of medication on academic achievement. As Aman (1993) observed, medication trials typically last 6–8 weeks, and it is difficult to assess the effects of medication on academic achievement in such a short period because most achievement tests are sluggish in picking up gains over a short period (R. T. Brown & Borden, 1989).

Analogue classroom tests are often used to assess academic productivity. They consist of numerous sheets containing arithmetic, spelling, or reading problems, similar to familiar classroom work sheets (Aman, 1993). Although the measures typically are not standardized, they include the number of problems that the child attempted as well as the number of problems that are correct (Aman, 1993; R. T. Brown & Sexson, 1988; R. T. Brown et al., 1991; Douglas et al., 1986; Handen, Breaux, Gosling, Ploof, & Feldman, 1990; Pelham, Bender, Caddell, Booth, & Moorer, 1985). Aman (1993) suggested that these measures typically reflect changes in children's motivation and attention span, and, as a result, demonstrate sensitivity to stimulant drug effects in a number of clinical drug trials (for review, see Brown et al., 1997). Whether analogue classroom tests actually detect increased academic skill performance is unclear, although they are easy to administer and thus are appropriate for the assessment of the effects of psychotropic medication on academic functioning.

MODEL ASSESSMENT APPROACH

Atkins and Pelham (1991) recommended a multivariate approach to assessing psychotropic drug response. This approach employs behavioral observations from teachers, parents, peers, and the children themselves across a variety of situations to provide optimal information about drug effectiveness. This excellent model developed for the use of psychostimulants seems appropriate for evaluating all psychotropic medications.

Barkley et al. (1988) and Gadow et al. (1991) delineated procedures to evaluate medications in the laboratory, and these procedures may also be useful in the clinical setting. The procedures include (1) the use of placebo controls and double-blind trials to mitigate the possibility of biases in both parental and teacher reports of behavior; (2) randomization of the order of dose to control for order effects; (3) the use of multiple assessment measures, including laboratory measures, teacher and parent ratings of behavioral symptoms, performance on academic tests, and evaluation within social domains; (4) assessment of functioning during peak drug response; and (5) systematic evaluation of adverse side effects during active medication and placebo administration. Barkley et al. (1993) and Varley and Trupin (1982) recommended that a double-blind trial of medication be the prototype of assessment in the clinical setting, thereby allowing for an objective evaluation of medication and adequate assessment of adverse side effects at home and at school.

Psychologists and pediatricians can collaborate productively on whether trials of psychotropic medication are successful and whether one particular dose is more effective than another in unstructured versus structured activities. Such collaboration requires systematic data collection by both professionals to provide a cost-effective evaluation, guided by a reliable assessment process, which can enhance treatment decisions as well as document the efficacy of particular medications.

PREDICTING RESPONSE TO PSYCHOTROPIC MEDICATION

Over the years, investigators have searched for measures and rating instruments that accurately predict a successful response to a particular psychotropic medication. Most of the investigations involving children and adolescents were conducted with stimulants. Some recent research demonstrates that children with ADHD and comorbid internalizing behavioral symptoms (e.g., anxiety) exhibit poorer response to stimulants (DuPaul, et al., 1994; Tannock, Ickowicz, & Schachar, 1995). The studies are significant as they suggest the importance of possible diagnostic subtypes of ADHD and hence the importance of careful diagnostic assessment of children. Buitelaar et al. (1995) examined factors that predict favorable stimulant drug response in children with ADHD. Some investigators found that children who were high in disinhibition (i.e., similar to the DSM-IV hyperactive–impulsive type) display a particularly favorable response to methylphenidate on measures of cognition, behavior, and compliance with adult directives (Beery, Quay, & Pelham, 1995; Wilkison, Kircher, McMahon, & Sloan, 1995). Interestingly, children who were classified as low in disinhibition (i.e., similar to the DSM-IV ADHD primarily inattentive type) responded favorably to operant techniques without the use of stimulant medication (Beery et al., 1995). These important investigations support subtyping and careful diagnosis as a way to clarify differential response to stimulants. Additional investigation is needed to foster more precise prescribing of stimulants for specific subtypes of ADHD. Unfortunately, there is a dearth of studies predicting children's response to other psychotropic medications. Until more definitive research is forthcoming, the most appropriate means of assessing drug response is the use of a systematic drug trial, after taking care to match the specific class of psychotropic to the child's target symptoms.

In a series of investigations, Barkley and colleagues (Barkley, 1991; Barkley & Grodzinsky, 1994; Barkley, Grodzinsky, & DuPaul, 1992) assessed the accuracy of various neurocognitive instruments in correctly classifying children as having symptoms of ADHD relative to their typically developing peers. They found little evidence to support the validity of widely used cognitive performance measures to identify children with ADHD. In understanding these results, readers should recognize that, for most externalizing disorders, symptom display is variable and contingent upon the demands and structure imposed by the environment (Barkley, 1990). Thus, in structured settings that characterize psychological evaluations, significant reinforcement is likely to be provided for on-task behavior. As a result, many children with externalizing disorders such as ADHD perform optimally. As a result, if psychologists rely solely on psychometric test data obtained in one-to-one settings to assess response to medication, false-negative or false-positive results may occur. For this reason, current standards of practice mandate that children be assessed across situational contexts (i.e., both at home and at school). Although the assessment of mental abilities, achievement, and cognitive skills is necessary to classify children as learning disabled or intellectually challenged, given the data presented by Barkley (Barkley, 1991; Barkley et al., 1992; DuPaul et al., 1992), testing should be interpreted judiciously in the assessment of drug response and should be used only in conjunction with a comprehensive history of development, objective school and home observation, and/or teacher and parent ratings of behavior.

CONCLUSIONS

Psychologists have an armamentarium of assessment techniques available to evaluate the behavioral and cognitive responses of children and adolescents to psychotropic medications. Medication response ideally should be evaluated across physical, behavioral, cognitive, and affective domains (Werry & Aman, 1993b). Despite the availability of an ideal prototype for a thorough medication evaluation, physicians do not always use objective data to guide decisions about titration of doses and treatment efficacy (Wolraich et al., 1990).

Behavioral assessment is the major approach used to evaluate children's response to medication and to monitor their progress. A variety of techniques are available to assess behavior, including direct observation, rating scales, and peer, or sociometric, ratings. Direct observations coupled with clearly delineated measures minimize observer interference and thus increase the objective measurement of responses (Atkins & Pelham, 1991). Observations should be conducted in a classroom or playroom, and observers should be blind as to the diagnosis and medication levels of the children being observed. Reliable and valid observational procedures have been successful in documenting stimulant drug effects. Rating scales provide a summary of behavior and offer several advantages, including simplicity, cost-effectiveness, and reduced subjectivity (Gadow, 1993a).

Perhaps the best model of assessment of efficacy and management of psychotropic medication is based on the voluminous studies on stimulant medication for children with ADHD. Direct observations of behavior and behavioral assessment techniques are hailed as the assessments of choice in evaluating children's responses to psychotropic medication in a number of areas of functioning. These approaches also have the advantage of evaluating behavioral domains with significant ecological validity (DuPaul & Kyle, 1995). Much more research is needed on the development of behavioral observations for other types of psychopathology so that response to other psychotropic medications can be appropriately and accurately measured.

Finally, the development of performance test instruments and computerized assessment techniques to evaluate drug response is an enterprising endeavor among test publishers. Psychological testing is merely one facet of a comprehensive test battery to evaluate a child for the possibility of a trial of medication, and psychological tests should always be used in conjunction with behavioral observations and teacher and parent ratings of behavior. A series of investigations evaluating the predictive power of a number of performance test instruments to assess psychopathology found that the level of sensitivity for the clinical groups was low; that is the measures did not adequately discriminate children with ADHD from their normal peers. Moreover, having a score on a cognitive task that falls within the normal range does not necessarily suggest the absence of psychopathology or learning problems. In fact, the behavioral and cognitive functioning of children and adolescents in a one-to-one testing situation and a traditional classroom setting may vary. Because the administration of these tests is often labor intensive and costly and the tests are of questionable ecological validity, their appropriateness for evaluating drug response must be carefully considered. No specific test instrument accurately predicts a positive response to medication. Thus, psychological test instruments are apt to be most helpful when used in conjunction with behavioral observations in the home environment (Barkley et al., 1988), classroom setting (Gadow, 1993a; Nolan & Gadow, 1994), and with peers (Pelham & Hoza, 1987).

Appendix A
STIMULANT DRUG SIDE EFFECTS RATING SCALE

Name _____ Date _____

Person Completing This Form _____

Instructions: Please rate each behavior from 0 (absent) to 9 (serious). Circle only one number beside each item. A zero means that you have not seen the behavior in this child during the past week, and a 9 means that you have noticed it and believe it to be either very serious or to occur very frequently.

Behavior	Absent									Serious
Insomnia or trouble sleeping	0	1	2	3	4	5	6	7	8	9
Nightmares	0	1	2	3	4	5	6	7	8	9
Stares a lot or daydreams	0	1	2	3	4	5	6	7	8	9
Talks less with others	0	1	2	3	4	5	6	7	8	9
Uninterested in others	0	1	2	3	4	5	6	7	8	9
Decreased appetite	0	1	2	3	4	5	6	7	8	9
Irritable	0	1	2	3	4	5	6	7	8	9
Stomachaches	0	1	2	3	4	5	6	7	8	9
Headaches	0	1	2	3	4	5	6	7	8	9
Drowsiness	0	1	2	3	4	5	6	7	8	9
Sad/unhappy	0	1	2	3	4	5	6	7	8	9
Prone to crying	0	1	2	3	4	5	6	7	8	9
Anxious	0	1	2	3	4	5	6	7	8	9
Bites fingernails	0	1	2	3	4	5	6	7	8	9
Euphoric/unusually happy	0	1	2	3	4	5	6	7	8	9
Dizziness	0	1	2	3	4	5	6	7	8	9
Tics or nervous movements	0	1	2	3	4	5	6	7	8	9

Appendix B
CHILDHOOD ATTENTION PROBLEMS RATING SCALE

Child's Name _____ Child's Age _____

Filled Out by _____ Child's Sex [ ] M [ ] F

Directions: Below is a list of items that describe pupils. For each item that describes the pupil now or within the past week, check whether the item is **Not True, Somewhat or Sometimes True,** or **Very or Often True.** Please check all items as well as you can, even if some do not seem to apply to this pupil.

	Not True	Somewhat or Sometimes True	Very or Often True
1. Fails to finish things he/she starts	[ ]	[ ]	[ ]
2. Can't concentrate, can't pay attention for long	[ ]	[ ]	[ ]
3. Can't sit still, restless, or hyperactive	[ ]	[ ]	[ ]
4. Fidgets	[ ]	[ ]	[ ]
5. Daydreams or gets lost in his/her thoughts	[ ]	[ ]	[ ]
6. Impulsive or acts without thinking	[ ]	[ ]	[ ]
7. Difficulty following directions	[ ]	[ ]	[ ]
8. Talks out of turn	[ ]	[ ]	[ ]
9. Messy work	[ ]	[ ]	[ ]
10. Inattentive, easily distracted	[ ]	[ ]	[ ]
11. Talks too much	[ ]	[ ]	[ ]
12. Fails to carry out assigned tasks	[ ]	[ ]	[ ]

Please feel free to write any comments about the pupil's work or behavior in the last week. _____

_____

_____

CHAPTER 7

◆◆◆

Acceptability and
Satisfaction Issues

◆

CONSUMER ATTITUDES AND SATISFACTION

The concept of treatment acceptability draws attention to the importance of attitudes held by parents and children about the appropriateness of a prescribed treatment (Kazdin, 1980, 1981, 1984). Negative attitudes may influence the initial willingness of children and parents to accept treatment and may also adversely affect the integrity of a psychopharmacological treatment program. The likelihood that a particular intervention will be fully adopted by children and parents may be constrained by popular beliefs about the availability of treatments, time and effort required for treatment implementation, and previous experience of treatment (Cross-Calvert & Johnston, 1990; Elliott, 1988). Thus, a key issue that must be addressed when pharmacological treatment for children and adolescents is being considered is the acceptability of the treatment to children, parents, and teachers.

Many parents and children are reluctant to use medications and may perceive pharmacotherapy as less acceptable or desirable than behavioral therapy (Kazdin, 1984; Summers & Caplan, 1987). As Barkley, Conners, et al. (1990) observed, there is often a preference for environmental management of school children's behavioral difficulties over psychopharmacological management. Investigators also suggest that drugs are less acceptable for use with children because of the difficulty of obtaining informed consent from children (for review, see R. T. Brown et al., in press). This issue is particularly relevant for psychologists who work with children and may be in a position to offer treatments other than medication. This issue also is similar to findings in the behavioral medicine literature, in which parents and caretakers are described as being more accepting of behavioral modalities for managing pain than they are of pain management involving analgesic medication (Tarnowski, Gavaghan, & Wisniewski, 1989). Because psychologists are particularly sensitive to developmental issues, they can play an important role in assisting children to understand the role of medication in the overall treatment program.

Behavioral techniques such as positive reinforcement, response cost, and time out are generally preferred over drug treatment (Kazdin, 1980, 1981, 1984; Kazdin, French, & Sherick, 1981). The severity of symptoms associated with the behavior disorders and the frequency of adverse side effects also influence medication acceptability (Kazdin, 1980, 1981, 1984). For example, in many cases, parents' and children's ratings of acceptability may differ markedly. This difference highlights the importance of carefully assessing both the child's and parents' attitudes when proposing a treatment plan that involves pharmacotherapy.

Unfortunately, most studies investigating treatment acceptability have focused only on alternatives for children with ADHD. In general, these studies were limited to comparing the relative acceptability of operant techniques to stimulant-drug therapy. There is scant research on the treatment acceptability of other psychotropic medications that are typically used with disorders for which there are more limited choices of alternative behavioral interventions. It is possible that the acceptability of drug treatment will be much greater in the latter situations.

Community Attitudes

Community attitudes about illegal and inappropriate prescribed drug use may influence decisions about the very medication to help schoolchildren with learning and behavioral problems. Although the use of psychotropic medication for adult psychopathology is widely accepted, the use of medication with children still tends to attract controversy (for review, see Gadow, 1993b). Opponents argue that conceptualizing children's social problems as diseases and then treating children with drugs fails to address the underlying causes of the problems (Barkley, Conners, et al., 1990). Some adherents of this position adopt the extreme view of comparing the use of psychotropic medication to slavery and child abuse (J. L. Brown & Bing, 1976). Others simply advocate for environmental management rather than the medical management of behavioral and learning problems experienced by children (Barkley, Conners, et al., 1990). Kazdin (1980) pointed out that society may view pharmacotherapy as unacceptable in managing problems for which equally effective environmental manipulations of behavior and learning were successful. Kazdin (1980) notes that "consumers are likely to be especially protective of children who are often not considered to be competent to weigh the manifold considerations (e.g., risks and benefits) that enter into treatment decisions" (p. 261).

Summers and Caplan (1987) used vignettes to assess lay beliefs about psychotropic medications for schoolchildren. They found that people tended to endorse the use of medication for disorders with an organic etiology. For example, in one vignette, a boy was described as walking around the classroom and disrupting the class during academic activities. In a second vignette, a boy was described as needing an anticonvulsant medication for a seizure disorder. Survey respondents indicated that the use of medication would be a more appropriate treatment modality for the child with a seizure disorder that was considered to be of organic etiology than for a disorder related to learning and behavior. The study also found that many respondents believed that psychotropic medication exacerbates psychological symptoms. Similarly, Mittle and Robin (1987), in their ratings of treatment acceptability for parent–adolescent conflict, found that undergraduate students rated medication as less acceptable than problem-solving communication and behavioral contracting; medication was rated ahead only of paradoxical therapy, which was found to be the least acceptable treatment modality for managing parent–adolescent conflict. Kazdin (1980, 1981, 1984) pointed out that medication is never rated as the most acceptable treatment when compared to other therapies, including behavior management.

Parental Attitudes

Varying parental attitudes about stimulant treatment may explain why parents differ in the consistency with which they administer medication to their children and why some parents discontinue medication prematurely (Cross-Calvert & Johnston, 1990). For example, Liu, Robin, Brenner, and Eastman (1991) surveyed mothers of children who were diagnosed with ADHD as well as those of nonreferred children about the relative acceptability of medication, behavior modification, and a combination in the management of ADHD. Despite reports of the medication's efficacy, both groups of parents rated behavior modification as more acceptable than stimulant medication. After several months of treatment, parents of children diagnosed with ADHD rated the combination of medication and behavioral therapy as superior to behavioral therapy alone. This finding suggests that greater parent knowledge of the disorder is related to greater acceptability of pharmacotherapy.

Slimmer and Brown (1985) studied the impact of a decision-making conference designed to facilitate treatment acceptance and reduce initial negative attitudes toward medication. Findings indicated that mothers' decisions showed more accepting attitudes about medication trials when they were able to express feelings of guilt about the disorder, consider all treatment alternatives, and rank treatment alternatives.

Finally, Borden and Brown (1989) examined the attributional effects of combining medication with psychotherapy in treating children with externalizing behavior disorders. All the children in their study received intensive cognitive therapy that emphasized self-control. In addition, all children were randomly assigned to methylphenidate, placebo, or a no-pill regimen. Parents of children in the no-pill condition more strongly believed that their children were capable of solving their own problems compared with parents of children in the placebo group, whereas parents of children on active medication and on placebo endorsed the efficacy of medication in assisting children with their behavioral problems. The placebo group most strongly believed that solutions would result from external and uncontrollable factors. Figure 7.1 presents the data. The results suggest medication may have important messages for parents.

In a recent study designed to assess the social importance and personal benefits associated with the participation in drug trials, Aman and Wolford (1995) surveyed parents of children with mental retardation who had participated in several drug trials. Parents were most satisfied when the efficacy of medication was evaluated in a systematic manner. This study is important because it draws attention to the capacity of double-blind trials to promote greater acceptance of medication use by parents.

Another study examined the relative acceptability of various treatments for internalizing disorders, including depression. In this study,

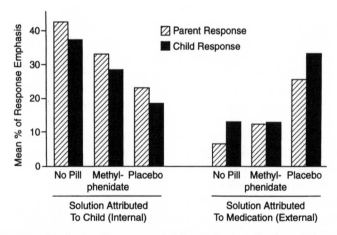

FIGURE 7.1. Similarity of parent and child attributions for the solution of child's presenting problems From Borden & Brown (1989). Copyright 1989 by Plenum Publishing Corp. Reprinted by permission.

Tarnowski, Simonian, Bekeny, and Park (1992) presented mothers of children referred for depression with vignettes that described children experiencing levels of depressive symptoms ranging from mild to severe. The mothers ranked pharmacological treatment as significantly less acceptable than all other treatments for both mild and severe depression, a finding consistent with mothers' discomfort with medication for behavioral disorders in childhood (e.g., oppositional defiant disorder, ADHD, conduct disorder). These data are consistent with those of Liu et al. (1991).

Werry and Aman (1993b) argued that although some parents may resist physicians' recommendations for drug treatment, others may view the recommendations as evidence that their child has an illness with a biological etiology rather than a disorder arising as a result of familial discord or maladaptive parenting. Clinicians need to be aware of the complex messages that a recommendation for medication treatment may convey to parents and families. Again, the psychologist can play an important role in clarifying these subtle and meaningful messages.

Teacher Attitudes

Many children receiving medication for behavior problems must receive doses during school hours. As a result, teachers' knowledge of and attitudes about pharmacological interventions are important. To date, research is limited almost entirely to studies of teachers' attitudes about psychopharmacological treatment for children with attention disturbances. Using a vignette, Epstein, Matson, Repp, and Helsel (1986) asked regular and special education teachers in training to rate the acceptability of treatments used to modify the ADHD symptoms of a first-grade boy. Treatment choices included medication, behavior modification, counseling, special education programming, and affective education. Both groups of teachers endorsed special education as the most appropriate treatment modality and indicated that medication was the least appropriate intervention. Kasten, Coury, and Heron (1992) also reported that more than 40% of special educators believed that too many students receive stimulants. Furthermore, 35% of the educators also thought that stimulants were prescribed too frequently for children diagnosed with ADHD. Similarly, Power, Hess, and Bennett (1995) reported that elementary and middle-school teachers rated behavioral interventions as more acceptable than stimulant drug therapy. Further, stimulant medication was rated as more acceptable when used in combination with behavior therapy than when used alone.

Such negative attitudes may not be surprising given Gadow's (1982) report that teachers were dismayed by the lack of communication between physicians and teachers about the medication status of children.

Other studies reported that special education teachers of seriously emotionally disturbed (Epstein, Singh, Luebke, & Stout, 1991) and learning disabled (Singh, Epstein, Luebke, & Singh, 1990) children believe that school personnel have little influence on decisions about whether or not medication should be used to manage disorders that affect children's academic performance or behavior at school. Most of the teachers indicated that they needed additional training in issues related to drug therapy for children. Both groups of teachers also said that the teachers' subjective anecdotal reports about medication effects were the most prevalent method of assessing treatment efficacy. However, the quality of these global impressions may be questionable as 86% of the teachers of learning-disabled pupils (Singh et al., 1990) and 95% of the teachers of seriously emotionally disturbed pupils (Epstein et al., 1991) indicated that they needed more training in issues related to drug treatment for children.

Finally, one investigation compared medication beliefs among mainstream educators, school psychologists, and special educators. In this study, Malyn, Jenson, and Clark (1993) asked how likely educators and psychologists would be to recommend stimulant medication to the parents of the children with ADHD with whom they worked. Although more than 80% of the school psychologists endorsed the efficacy of stimulant medication for children with ADHD, only one third indicated that they would inform parents about stimulant treatment, versus 55% of regular and special educators.

Child and Peer Attitudes

A large number of studies have investigated children's attitudes and expectations about pharmacotherapy. Because many psychotropic medications require multiple doses throughout the day, children frequently receive medication while at school, and often in front of their peers. Knowledge by other children that a child with ADHD is receiving medication may further affect the social relations of children with ADHD (Whalen & Henker, 1991b). In fact, because most stimulant treatment regimens for ADHD involve a noontime dose at school, this treatment may have greater potential than other forms of intervention to stigmatize children with ADHD. This finding is of major concern because children with ADHD are known to be at risk for problems with peers (Landau & Moore, 1991). This hypothesis was investigated by Sigelman and Shorokey (1986), who examined children's attributions and the relative likability of a hypothetical child described as hyperactive ("always on the go") who either received pharmacological therapy or exerted personal effort to control problem behavior in the classroom. Results indicated that the boy was more likable when good management of his problem was perceived to be based on effort rather than on medication. However, Sigelman and Shorokey (1986) found that the respondents' grade level in school also affected their views of pharmacological treatment. Specifically, the management approach mattered to fourth- and fifth-grade children only when the child in the vignette achieved success; for kindergarten and first-grade children, the type of solution mattered only if the treatment failed. Thus, younger children's acceptance of the boys was not diminished by medication status as long as it worked. These findings support the developmental nature of children's attributional analyses (see also Amirkhan, 1982), and, most important, provide preliminary data to suggest that children's knowledge of the medication status of a child with ADHD may affect the child's social status.

Even though school personnel can take steps to ensure the confidentiality of a child's medication treatment, there is concern that cognitive and affective consequences may accrue for the child who receives pharmacological intervention (Whalen & Henker, 1976). Whalen and Henker and their associates (Henker & Whalen, 1989; Whalen & Henker, 1976; Whalen, Henker, Hinshaw, Heller, & Huber-Dressler, 1991) argued that pharmacological treatment for ADHD may lead to iatrogenic effects, as medication use may convey an undesirable message to the child about personal control and competence. For example, stimulant treatment for ADHD may cause a child to attribute improved behavior to an external cause (the medication) while rendering the child's efforts and capabilities irrelevant (in the child's eyes) to improved performance at school (Henker & Whalen, 1989). This diminished sense of self-efficacy may intrude on the child's persistence with future learning tasks and academic achievement. In other words, children may consider their efforts and capabilities to be impotent, thereby further impeding their learning.

The most definitive work on this issue was presented by Milich and Pelham and their colleagues (C. L. Carlson, Pelham, Milich, & Hoza, 1993; Milich, Carlson, Pelham, & Licht, 1991; Pelham, Murphy, et al., 1992). In this series of well-controlled laboratory investigations, boys with ADHD were exposed to success and failure conditions in a counterbalanced medication and placebo trial. Medication appeared to exert a differential effect on performance, where it enhanced persistence but only in the face of failure. In addition, when attributions for success and failure were examined, boys receiving active medication did not differ in their attributions following exposure to solvable tasks compared to boys who received placebo. However, following failure, medicated boys made significantly more external (i.e., task difficulty) and significantly fewer internal (i.e., effort) attributions on medication versus placebo. Thus, the use of medication diminished the boys' sense of personal responsibility for failure, a pattern consistent with a more adaptive and healthy response style

(S. E. Taylor & Brown, 1988). Pelham, Murphy, et al. (1992) replicated this investigation with the addition of a no-pill experimental condition. They found that children receiving medication attributed success to their ability or effort and attributed failure to the medication or program staff.

Contrary to predictions of undesirable iatrogenic effects (Whalen & Henker, 1991b), the studies by C. L. Carlson et al. (1993) and Milich et al. (1991b) suggested that medicated boys with ADHD did not blame themselves when faced with failure. Instead, they attributed their lack of success to the difficulties inherent in the task. In addition, a study reported by Milich et al. (1989) found that boys with ADHD were significantly more accurate in assessing the quality of their vigilance on a task of sustained attention when on medication than when on placebo. Taken together, these findings indicate that medication may permit boys with ADHD to function more like mastery-oriented children, who are capable of accurately evaluating their own performance (Dweck & Leggett, 1988). The performance of unmedicated children with ADHD, on the other hand, may be more like those who have a helplessness orientation (Milich, 1994). Consistent with this, N. J. Cohen and Thompson (1982) found that most children with ADHD believed they had greater internal control while on medication, and two thirds indicated a desire to continue the regimen if given the choice. This finding is corroborated by Bowen, Fenton, and Rappaport (1991), who found that the majority of children who were being treated with stimulants reported the treatment helpful.

In a more recent investigation, Ialongo, Lopez, Horn, Pascoe, and Greenberg (1994) investigated the effects of stimulant medication on children's ratings of self-competence. No diminished perceptions of competence were reported by the children. Milich et al. (1989) found that boys with ADHD who were receiving stimulant medication were more accurate in assessing the quality of their vigilance performance on a task of sustained attention. Thus, children who received stimulant medication behaved in a mastery-oriented fashion, whereby they were accurate in assessing their own performance. Their unmedicated peers with ADHD displayed helplessness.

There is a paucity of research investigating peer and child attitudes about psychopharmacological interventions of children's learning and behavior disorders. More research on treatment acceptability and on the adverse effects of psychotropic medications on peer group attitudes is particularly needed for psychotropic medications other than stimulants.

Attitudes of Health Care Providers

Werry and Aman (1993b) underscored some important principles that affect the decision to prescribe medication. First, the investigators emphasized that the empirical literature to date, particularly with pediatric populations, is atheoretical. Few guidelines exist to determine whether a particular medication is likely to be safe and effective for an individual child with a behavioral or learning problem. Thus, the current state of medical knowledge is quite primitive, and often the only way to determine whether a medication will be efficacious and safe for any particular child is to try it. This requires that every drug trial proceed with careful assessment and the utmost caution to document safety and efficacy.

An important issue related to assessing safety and efficacy is the "placebo effect," whereby both caretakers and physicians perceive a positive medication effect that is not supported by more objective data and rigorous trials. For example, Sulzbacher (1973) analyzed both double-blind placebo-controlled trials and trials that did not use placebo and found that investigations that did not use placebos reported higher success rates than those that did use placebos. This analysis underscores the importance of using objective data and rigorous trials to quantify drug efficacy and safety.

Most health care providers want to be helpful to their patients and at the same time earn a living in a field that is becoming more difficult because of marked changes in the U.S. health care system. As a result, financial issues can impinge on decisions about whether or not to use psychopharmacotherapy for children (Werry & Aman, 1993b). Health care providers must be cognizant of such subtle influences on their prescribing patterns. An important influence on physicians' attitudes may be advertising by the pharmaceutical industry. As Werry and Aman (1993b) point out, pharmaceutical companies invest millions of dollars in advertising, which is ubiquitous in clinic and hospital settings and in the pages of most medical journals. One possible impact of advertising is that, although generic brands are cheaper than brand-name drugs, brand-name drugs may continue to be prescribed.

Summary

In the community, medication is generally rated less favorably than psychotherapies and behavioral approaches. However, parents are likely to be more willing to medicate their child when a systematic drug trial documenting efficacy and any adverse side effects was conducted. Teachers' attitudes are similar to parental attitudes and can also be modified by providing teachers with greater input about the medication process. As studies of the long-term effects of various psychotropics confirm both the efficacy and safety of psychotropics, the attitudes of teachers and parents may shift. However, children's attitudes about psychotropic medication may be very different from those of their caretakers and teachers. It is essential that clinicians evaluate the attitudes of all the people in a child's environment who are affected by a drug treatment program, including parents, teachers, and children. Finally, health care providers have definite attitudes about psychotropic medication, yet they are frequently ignored in both the clinical and empirical literature. A host of issues need to be considered, including providers' knowledge and education about drugs, possible economic gains, and unrealistic expectations in efforts to assist parents and children with their difficulties.

COMPLIANCE

Compliance can be divided into attrition (the premature discontinuation of treatment) and the alteration of drug administration procedures during treatment (e.g., increasing or decreasing the dose level). Both are common among pediatric patients, even children of the most well-intentioned parents. When psychotropic medication is the drug being administered, compliance problems increase exponentially (for review, see R. T. Brown et al., in press).

Placing any child on psychotropic medication is a decision that must be weighed carefully and must be based on a thorough evaluation with clearly delineated target behaviors and treatment goals. To maximize the likelihood of success, professionals treating the child should follow a collaborative team model that includes clear and direct communication among team members and parents (Roberts, 1986).

When a child takes medication, it is important to provide education about the medication and its associated benefits and adverse side effects. Parents are responsible for making decisions about their children and must provide consent before pharmacotherapy is initiated; assent should also be obtained from children. Health care providers must be sensitive to cultural issues that may influence values, expectations, and norms about psychopathology and medication (Westermeyer, 1987).

Because psychotropics may be administered for long periods and because parents and children are often ambivalent about medication, compliance problems increase over time (Cross-Calvert & Johnston, 1990; Johnston & Fine, 1993; Tarnowski, Kelly, & Mendlowitz, 1987). Parents' concerns about the use of medication for children may result in pharmacotherapy being underutilized despite compelling evidence that medications can be highly beneficial in the symptom management of several childhood disorders. As medicines often have to be administered at school, compliance may be affected by school staff members' attitudes toward medications.

Many studies suggest that children and parents fail to adhere to prescribed medical regimens and may eventually discontinue treatment prematurely (R. T. Brown et al., 1987; Firestone, 1982; Kauffman, Smith-Wright, Reese, Simpson, & Fowler, 1981). For example, in a study by R. T. Brown et al. (1987) in which compliance was verified by pharmacist counts, nearly one fourth of prescribed stimulant medication was not taken. Rates of compliance were directly associated with social class and intellectual functioning, with children from higher socioeconomic backgrounds and more intelligent parents being more compliant.

Firestone (1982) reported that nearly 20% of subjects in a study of children receiving medication discontinued the medication prematurely within 4 months and fewer than 10% of parents consulted with project staff before discontinuing their children's medication. By 10 months, nearly 50% of children had discontinued their medication. Parents indicated that adverse effects often were their primary reason for discontinuing medication prematurely. Further, the more numerous the adverse side effects, the more likely the noncompliance (DuPaul & Kyle, 1995; LaGreca & Schulman, 1995). Using urine screens, Kauffman et al. (1981) found that one third of children in a study of hyperactive boys did not adhere to prescribed drug regimens in any given week. Zametkin and Yamada (1993) argued that noncompliance with treatment is a major reason for the failure of children to respond to drug treatment programs.

Johnston and Fine (1993) suggested that acceptability, satisfaction, and compliance with treatment are intricately related. As R. T. Brown and Borden (1989) observed, numerous factors influence these issues, including the need for long-term treatment, negative publicity in the lay press, and fears about the adverse side effects of psychotropic medication. Brown and Borden described the long course of treatment for children with behavior and learning disorders as being analogous to a learned-helplessness phenomenon in which parents are unable to envision meeting hoped-for goals within a reasonable time and, as a result, perceive that they have little control over their child's symptoms. Brown and Borden suggested that the use of medication to manage children's problems may communicate to family members that a child's symptoms are out of the child's or family's control. Thus, the belief in an inability to effect improvements may compound a family's demoralization in response to having a child with a major learning or behavior disorder.

In an effort to investigate the relationship among treatment acceptability, satisfaction, and compliance, Johnston and Fine (1993) compared two treatment approaches. One approach used a double-blind drug trial and the other a standard evaluation of drug efficacy. Children with ADHD were assigned randomly either to a controlled double-blind medication trial or to a clinical evaluation that was nonblind and lacked placebo controls. The investigators found that ratings of treatment satisfaction were higher among parents whose child participated in the double-blind drug trial, although all parents' acceptance of stimulant medication showed improvement. However, consistent with previous studies of adherence (R. T. Brown et al., 1987; Firestone, 1982; Kauffman et al., 1981), Johnston and Fine (1993) found that approximately one fifth of the sample was noncompliant at both 6-week and 3-month follow-ups. Thus, although no differences were found for rates of adherence between the two treatment groups, the study suggests that good-quality clinical drug trials may enhance treatment and consumer satisfaction. The investigation is important, as it supports a positive correlation between patient education (such as reviewing potential benefits and adverse side effects with parents and children) and treatment satisfaction.

The investigation by Johnston and Fine (1993) demonstrated that developing therapeutic rapport and providing support to parents and children can assist with patient satisfaction. Parents and children must be provided with adequate information about medication and appropriate strategies to overcome obstacles that will hinder compliance with the medication. Adherence must also be carefully assessed before reaching conclusions about either the short- or long-term efficacy of treatment with any medication. For example, it is possible that the poor long-term outcomes reflect a failure of children and families to adhere to prescribed drug treatment procedures rather than inherent limitations of the medication (R. T. Brown & Borden, 1989; Sleator, 1985).

The importance of family support for children's treatment adherence is underscored in the pediatric psychology literature (LaGreca & Schulman, 1995). Other factors associated with positive medication adherence include peer support, simplifying treatment regimens, structuring medication administration, and providing rewards for appropriate adherence. Adherence with medication regimens is a complex issue, and clinicians need to assess compliance carefully before evaluating either the short- or long-term efficacy of any medication used to improve learning and behavior.

In summary, when interventions are unacceptable to parents, satisfaction and compliance with treatment are at risk (Cross-Calvert & Johnston, 1990; Tarnowski, et al., 1987). Parental and teacher concerns may mean that medications will be underutilized for children who might benefit from their use. In addition, children and their parents may fail to adhere to the prescribed regimen of the medication or may prematurely discontinue treatment. School personnel can be actively involved in assisting parents and children with medication compliance, regardless of whether the medication is administered at school. Many psychotropic medications must be administered during the course of the schoolday, and the attitudes and availability of school staff may affect compliance and treatment acceptability (R. T. Brown et al., 1994).

ETHICAL ISSUES

Barkley, Conners, et al. (1990) highlighted a range of ethical issues that must be addressed when psychotropic medications are prescribed for pediatric populations. As with many ethical problems, there is no straightforward answer to many of these issues. Nonetheless, each issue deserves careful evaluation in terms of risks and benefits. When psychologists either participate in the recommendation to provide medication to treat a child's problem or engage in the assessment of efficacy or adverse side effects, the following must be addressed:

1. The extent to which adults should be the focus of treatment, rather than the child, as children do not initiate psychiatric treatment.
2. Ethical issues about the widespread use of these agents with children and adolescents, because the long-term effects of most psychotropic agents are not well understood for children and adolescents who are undergoing rapid physical development and brain growth.
3. The increased use of therapies that emphasize a biological approach to manage children's behavior may result in a shift away from environmental variables and result in an exclusive focus on biological foundations of behavior.
4. Questions concerning the extent to which psychotropic medications alter children's locus of control, self-efficacy, and motivation.
5. Concerns that medications may be overprescribed because they are more convenient than the psychotherapies and special education programs.
6. The limited ability of children suffering from learning and behavioral problems to provide self-reports about mood and adverse side effects associated with psychotropic medication, acknowledging that psychotropic medication may mask some of the difficulties in the life circumstances of children and adolescents.
7. The lack of sufficient empirical data about the efficacy and safety of psychotropic agents for pediatric populations to justify their widespread use.

LEGAL ISSUES AND INFORMED CONSENT

As with any medical treatment, there are laws in the United States and in most other countries designed to protect consumers. Although the scope of this chapter does not permit a full review of all of the legal issues involved in the provision of health care, psychologists should be familiar with legislation relevant to the prescribing of medication for children. This is important because psychologists are often involved in assessing the safety and efficacy of medications used by children with various learning and behavioral disorders.

Informed consent is a major issue that embraces both the ethical and legal principles guiding the practice of all health care providers. Informed consent pertaining to psychotropic medication requires that the prescribing physician inform the patient of both the novelty of a new pharmaceutical and any possible unknown, as well as documented, adverse side effects (Krener & Mancina, 1994; Nurcombe & Parlett, 1994). Potential risks, as well as alternative treatments, should be explained when psychotropics for children and adolescents are prescribed. Moreover, parents should be informed that unknown adverse effects of many medications may not appear until several years following termination of treatment. It is important to remember that parents or legal guardians, not the children and adolescents, hold privilege and, therefore, must provide informed consent. Schouten and Duckworth (1993) further caution physicians that, in most jurisdictions, the failure to obtain consent from a parent or guardian leaves physicians open to charges of malpractice and even battery. It is also essential, however, that children give assent for medication as a means of fostering a therapeutic alliance and encouraging some autonomy and responsibility with the medication regimen (Krener & Mancina, 1994; Schouten & Duckworth, 1993). Krener and Mancina suggested that failing to include the child or adolescent in the consent process causes feelings of coercion and may run counter to the therapeutic goals of treatment and the developmental interests of the child.

The issue of informed consent is particularly critical when prescribing antipsychotic medication (for review, see Schouten & Duckworth, 1993). Discussion with the parents or guardians should address the likelihood of tardive dyskinesia, alternative medications that might be useful, the potential irreversibility of dyskinesias, and a risk-benefit analysis of the use of this class of drugs with a child or adolescent.

Informed consent also requires that the patient's decision to accept medication is voluntary and without coercion (Krener & Mancina, 1994). In the treatment of children, it is the parents or guardian who hold privilege, and these individuals should accept treatment on the child's behalf voluntarily and free of coercion. A physician or psychologist who coerces a patient into consenting to any treatment may be subject to charges of battery (Schouten & Duckworth, 1993). Although it is legal and possibly ethical for parents to coerce a child or adolescent into a specific treatment, a physician or psychologist must not engage in such practice.

Schouten and Duckworth (1993) also recommended documentation of informed consent, either formal or informal. Documentation should include: (1) topics discussed, (2) individuals present, (3) a listing of risks and benefits, (4) questions raised, (5) subsequent consent, and (6) evidence that an opportunity was provided to ask further questions.

Informed consent requires that the individual be competent to provide consent. Schouten and Duckworth (1993) argue that an individual is competent if the following criteria are met: (1) the individual has attained a factual understanding of the situation that includes the needs and alternatives involved, (2) the individual understands the potential seriousness of the condition and the consequences of accepting or rejecting treatment, and (3) the individual can express a preference and manipulate the information provided in a rational manner.

A final issue relates to parental custody. Frequently, a child whose parents are separated or divorced may be in treatment and issues arise as to who may consent for treatment. As with the provision of any psychological services, it is the custodial parent who must provide informed consent. This issue may become more complex when both parents have custody and one parent objects to psychotropic medication. In this case, the physician must work carefully with both parents to achieve the best treatment for the child.

In providing psychological services and psychopharmacotherapy, as is the case with any psychotherapeutic relationship, confidentiality is the responsibility of the health care provider. However, because children are presumed not to be competent to provide consent, information must be shared with the child's parent or guardian in accordance with state law. Of course, it is the child's parent or guardian who will administer and monitor the medication, although school personnel also often become involved in the medication regimens. Thus, it is important to secure the trust of the parents and the child in obtaining consent to work collaboratively in contacting appropriate school personnel such as teachers and school nurses. In this way, school personnel may participate in the medication administration and the monitoring of behavior and cognition if medication is needed during school hours. This will ensure that the child attains maximum benefit and that adverse side effects of any medication are recognized and minimized.

Risk Management

Schouten and Duckworth (1993) delineated four elements that constitute justification for malpractice: (1) the psychologist or psychiatrist owed the patient a standard of care; (2) the psychologist or psychiatrist either failed to follow standard of practice or improperly applied standard of care; (3) the negligent behavior was the proximate (a legal concept that is an attempt to determine whether a particular event caused another event) cause of a particular injury; and, finally, (4) the negligent behavior resulted in damages that can be proven.

Written documentation of the child's history, mental status examination, current symptoms, treatment plan, risk–benefit analysis, and informed consent is essential during the course of treatment (Schouten & Duckworth, 1993). Schouten and Duckworth recommend that psychologists and other mental health providers consult with colleagues on a regular basis to obtain additional expertise and to reach consensus about the standard of care appropriate for particular disorders. They also recommend that practitioners avoid making promises guaranteeing a particular outcome that may leave the psychologist vulnerable for violation of a contract. Finally, they recommend that clinicians apologize for adverse events but caution against presenting themselves as responsible because this may not hold favorably in any future legal proceedings.

Summary

The use of pharmacotherapy with pediatric populations involves issues that are similar to the standard practice of psychotherapy with pediatric populations and their families but may require novel approaches. For example, detailing to a child's caretakers what is known and not known about a particular psychotropic necessitates distinctive knowledge and skill on the part of the practitioner. Good communication is also important so that parents of children are fully informed when they give their consent to treatment. Issues also emerge about competence to make decisions and refusing treatment. These issues become particularly thorny when parents disagree or when children refuse to take prescribed medication after their parents consented to this treatment. In such cases, excellent clinical skills, the capacity to address parents' concerns and negotiate with family members, and knowledge of appropriate legislation will serve the best interest of the child.

SOCIAL, POLITICAL, AND CULTURAL ISSUES

Children from lower socioeconomic backgrounds may be recommended for medication more frequently, whereas their peers from more affluent backgrounds may receive more costly psychotherapies or special education services, either as an adjunct or in lieu of psychotropic medication (Barkley, Conners, et al., 1990). There is a dearth of research related to safety and efficacy of psychotropic medication with specific racial and ethnic groups. To remedy this, situation, the National Institutes of Health mandated that national sampling for medical research should include 19% of underrepresented ethnic groups and a more equitable proportion of women or girls. Only one study could be identified that examined differential response in children as a function of race or ethnicity (R. T. Brown & Sexson, 1988).

There are compelling data about unique adverse side effects of certain psychotropic agents that are experienced by various racial and ethnic groups. For example, Strickland, Lin, Fu, Anderson, and Zheng (1995) found that African Americans experienced greater toxicities and other adverse side effects from treatment with lithium carbonate for the management of bipolar disorder than did those individuals of European descent. Similarly, for patients from Taiwan with bipolar disorder, Yang (1985) reported more favorable response with lower doses of lithium carbonate than was reported for individuals from European descent.

Some important data also suggest that tricyclic antidepressants are metabolized more slowly by Asian Americans than by other ethnic groups (Rudorfer & Robins, 1982). For example, Asians with severe depressive disorders were found to respond more positively to lower doses of combined imipramine and desipramine than those individuals of European descent (Flaskerud & Hu, 1994). Moreover, African Americans are at greater risk for toxicities and CNS effects with tricyclic antidepressants than are Asians, Latinos, and European Americans; one explanation may be the higher levels of absorption of antidepressants among the African American group (Rudorfer & Robins, 1982). Turkkan (1995) provided data to indicate that older African American women are more likely to display a higher side-effect profile with tricyclic antidepressants than were their European American counterparts.

Some research indicates that the anxiolytic drugs such as diazepam are metabolized more slowly by Asians than by Europeans or European Americans. For example, Asians are at higher risk than either Europeans or European Americans for toxicity to benzodiazepines administered either orally or intravenously (Fang, Hinrichs, & Ghoneim, 1987; Zhang, Reviriego, Lou, Sjoqvist, & Bertilsson, 1990).

All these studies suggest there may be unique issues pertaining to benefits, adverse side effects, and dose response of particular psychotropic agents for specific racial and ethnic groups. Representation among various racial and ethnic groups in future clinical trials with children will be important in determining whether there is, in fact, unique response as a function of both race and ethnicity.

Finally, for children with learning and behavior disorders from racial and ethnic groups who have comorbidity of other medical conditions, such as hypertension (which is prevalent among African Americans), further studies should carefully evaluate the potential benefits of any psychotropic medications with the adverse side effects that may be exacerbated by a specific medical condition. For example, R. T. Brown and Sexson (1988) demonstrated that hypertension is a particular adverse side effect of stimulant medication used for African American youngsters with ADHD.

CONCLUSIONS

Attitudes of society at large, as well as of parents, teachers, and health care providers, have important implications for treatment satisfaction and compliance with pharmacological regimens. Data suggest that when pharmacotherapy is pitted against any of the psychotherapies, medication is the least acceptable treatment modality. Attitudes among health care providers are important as there are scant data regarding the safety and efficacy, particularly in the longer term, of psychotropics for children and adolescents. Important placebo effects exist, and for this reason, careful objective monitoring is needed when prescribing psychotropics for children. The economic issues associated with managed care and the pharmaceutical industry may have a significant influence on prescribing practices by health-care providers working with children and adolescents.

School staff are an important influence shaping children's attitudes about medication and ensuring that medication is administered properly during the day. It is important for school psychologists to have training in psychopharmacology, including how specific psychotropics effect cognition, learning, and behavior. In addition, physicians need to sustain ongoing liaisons with psychologists in assisting with the monitoring of drug efficacy and with documenting any adverse cognitive and behavioral toxicities of specific psychotropics.

A host of ethical and legal considerations emerge when psychotropic agents are used to treat children and adolescents. These include conflicts associated with the drugs' administration because of the dearth of data addressing long-term safety and efficacy and the concern that medication may replace psychotherapy and special education because it is more cost-effective in the short term (but not necessarily more effective). As with any medical therapy, a number of issues involve liability, including informed consent, the right to refuse treatment, issues of custody, and, as in any therapeutic relationship, confidentiality. Careful risk management that includes systematic documentation, consultation with colleagues, and making realistic promises to children and their families is necessary.

Finally, as in other areas of psychology, social and cultural influences are likely to mediate children's and adolescents' attitudes, compliance, and possible responses to psychotropic medications. Cultural aspects of medication use receive far too little attention in both the adult and pediatric literatures. The study of ethnicity and pediatric psychopharmacology is another area in which psychologists can make a viable contribution to the empirical literature.

CHAPTER 8

♦♦♦

Issues Related to Training and Research

♦

As providers of mental health services to schoolchildren, psychologists are frequently called on to deliver diagnostic and therapeutic services to children and adolescents who are either receiving or being considered for a trial of psychotropic medication. Psychologists must understand both the direct effects of various agents on learning and behavior and the interaction of these pharmacotherapies with various types of psychoeducational and psychosocial therapies. Given their scientist–practitioner training, psychologists can bring significant research rigor to the field of pediatric psychopharmacology. Further, the fields of clinical, school, and counseling psychology have recently recognized that only treatments that have withstood the rigors of valid empirical research should be prescribed. With further training during both the pre- and postdoctoral years, psychologists can contribute significantly to the research on the myriad psychopharmacotherapies used with children and adolescents. As a result, a sound empirical foundation will be laid for the clinical practice of prescribing psychotropic agents for pediatric populations.

The issue of initiating prescribing privileges for psychologists has received widespread attention, particularly from those who train psychologists in a wide range of specializations, including clinical child psychologists (Barkley, Conners, et al., 1990) and school psychologists (C. L. Carlson & Kubiszyn, 1994). We encourage readers to examine some of the published articles on this topic (Adams & Bielauskas, 1994; Barkley et al., 1990; Burns, DeLeon, Chemtob, & Welch, in press; DeLeon, Folen, Jennings, Willis, & Wright, 1991; DeLeon, Fox, & Graham, 1991; DeLeon, Sammons, & Sexton, 1995; Frank, 1992; Piotrowski & Keller, 1996; Sammons, 1994). Many of our colleagues oppose the idea of prescribing privileges for psychologists (Adams & Bielauskas, 1994; Kratochowill, 1994). Others believe that such authority would enhance the status of psychologists in the provision of health care services and expand the role of psychology within the delivery of services, allowing the profession to have greater control over its own destiny (Burns et al., in press; DeLeon, Folen, et al., 1991; DeLeon, Fox, & Graham, 1991; DeLeon et al., 1995; Frank, 1992; Sammons, 1994). Still others (Barkley, Conners, et al., 1990) take a more neutral position, urging that psychologists consider all the ethical issues associated with the administration of psychotropics. In the end, we hope the ultimate decision about prescribing privileges will be based on the benefits the children and the families, rather than on issues pertaining to financial gain and social equality of psychologists with other health care providers.

Regardless of whether psychologists pursue the right to prescribe within a limited formulary, as Barkely, Conners, et al. (1990) observed, many already collaborate with pediatricians in decisions to medicate children. This collaboration may include a psychological evaluation documenting the presence of attentional problems that warrant a trial of a stimulant medication or proposing of a trial of medication to manage symptoms of depression. In lieu of this type of collaboration, graduate training for psychologists who work with pediatric populations should include a basic course in pediatric psychopharmacology. Because so many children receive psychotropics, it is important for psychologists to have training in understanding the clinical effects of these agents, particularly as they affect learning and behavior. The existing graduate curriculum also should be augmented to include monitoring of medication response, assessment of adverse side effects, and ethical issues associated with pharmacotherapy of children and adolescents. Further, traditional courses in assessment and ethics should be expanded to address appropriate psychopharmacotherapies for specific childhood disorders, as well as the assessment of medication response. These components also should be included in pre- and postdoctoral internship training programs to provide opportunities for collaboration with other health care providers in the area of psychopharmacology, with ample opportunities for supervision. Opportunities for continuing education and supervision should be available for psychologists who completed their doctoral training.

CURRICULUM

Of all the curricula proposed for practicing psychologists who might prescribe psychotropic medication (Ax & Babcock, 1995; Balster, 1990; Fox, Schwelitz, & Barclay, 1992), the most rigorous and inclusive is the curriculum proposed by the American Psychological Association (APA; 1996) for postdoctoral training in psychopharmacology. This curriculum is based, in part, on the Department of Defense demonstration project curriculum and the report of the Blue Ribbon Panel of the Professional Education Task Force of the California Psychological Association and the California School of Professional Psychology–Los Angeles, as well as the findings of the American College of Neuropsychopharmacology. Although the training program initially was conceived as a postdoctoral experience for practitioners already in the field, the curriculum also could be incorporated into a predoctoral program.

The purpose of the curriculum is to extend the traditional training in psychology to psychopharmacology within the context of several complex factors influencing human psychology (e.g., biological, environmental, interpersonal, behavioral, cognitive, emotional, motivational, psychosocial, and dynamic factors) (APA, 1996). The curriculum emphasizes integration of research and practice, focusing on the relationship between psychopharmacological and psychotherapeutic or psychoeducational interventions. In short, although psychopharmacology training must incorporate aspects of training from medicine, pharmacy, and nursing, it should be consistent with training in psychology that focuses on behavior and coping skills. Because the program builds its foundation on psychology, the training is unique to the needs of the practicing psychologist and does not emulate traditional medical practices.

The training model proposed by the APA (1996) includes both an emphasis on the requisite knowledge in psychopharmacology and the scientific methods and data on which this knowledge is based. In essence, the training model in psychopharmacology builds on the current training of psychologists in the scientific foundations of psychological practice. As delineated by the APA, an important goal is to prepare psychologists to evaluate new advances in psychopharmacology research and to prepare them for lifelong learning in the field that is destined to undergo significant transformation during their years of clinical practice.

Prerequisites for postdoctoral training should include the following: (1) a doctoral degree in psychology (i.e., PhD, PsyD, or EdD), (2) a current state license as a psychologist, and (3) practice as a "health-services provider" psychologist as defined by state law where applicable or as defined by the APA (1996).

Demonstrated knowledge of human biology, anatomy and physiology, biochemistry, neuroanatomy, and psychopharmacology is a necessary prerequisite for beginning postdoctoral-level training (APA, 1996). This demonstrated knowledge should include (1) evidence of successful completion of a planned sequence of courses at a regionally accredited institution of higher learning, or (2) evidence of successful completion of a planned sequence of continuing education courses offered by an accredited institution of higher learning or an approved provider of continuing education, and (3) passage of an examination covering the content of such programs. Individuals who are licensed health professionals with comparable prescription privileges in another profession and who are also licensed psychologists may be exempt from these training requirements by state boards of psychology.

According to the APA (1996), the courses and practica should be part of an organized and coordinated program of instruction. The APA intends that the program will develop admissions standards, including required prerequisite knowledge and a means of evaluating that knowledge. The program will allow credit for previous training and transfer of credit for previous course work.

The program will have appropriate faculty and facilities for the required didactic and clinical components of training. To provide the scope of training necessary, faculty with terminal degrees and expertise in the following disciplines is needed: physiology, biochemistry, neurosciences, pharmacology, psychology, pharmacy, medicine, and psychiatry (APA, 1996). The model mandates that didactic courses be administered for academic credit with careful attention to trainee evaluation. Students are required to meet levels of criterion-related performance. Finally, the providers of this training program must be regionally accredited institutions of higher learning or other appropriately accredited providers of instruction and training.

The APA (1996) recommends that a minimum of 300 contact hours of didactic instruction be distributed across the following core content areas:

I. Neurosciences
II. Pharmacology and Psychopharmacology
III. Physiology and Pathophysiology
IV. Physical and Laboratory Assessment
V. Clinical Pharmacotherapeutics

Recommended contact hours in each area are as follows:

Topic	Hours
I. Neurosciences	
A. Neuroanatomy	25
B. Neurophysiology	25
C. Neurochemistry	25
II. Clinical and Research Pharmacology and Psychopharmacology	
A. Pharmacology	30

Topic	Hours
B. Clinical Pharmacology	30
C. Psychopharmacology	45
D. Developmental Psychopharmacology	10
E. Chemical Dependency and Chronic Pain Management	15
III. Physiology and Pathophysiology	60

Pathophysiology should include normal anatomy and physiological processes in addition to common pathological states, with particular emphasis on how alterations in cardiovascular, renal, hepatic, gastrointestinal, neural, and endocrine functions affect bioavailability and biodisposition of drugs. This area also should address variability in drug bioavailability and biodisposition due to ethnic and cultural differences (APA, 1996). The APA (1996) recommends that the course include normal human anatomy and physiology as well as common pathological conditions that impact the safety and efficacy of various psychopharmacological agents. Variability in response due to age, gender, disability, and ethnic differences should be addressed. Finally, medical conditions affecting drug biodisposition and the likelihood of adverse side effects, including contraindications for medical use, also should be a component of coursework.

Topic	Hours
IV. Physical and Laboratory Assessment	45
(This would include familiarity with medical charts, physical examinations, laboratory, and radiological examinations.)	
V. Clinical Pharmacotherapeutics	
A. Professional, Ethical, and Legal Issues	10
B. Psychotherapy/Pharmacotherapy Interactions	10
C. Computer-Based Aids to Practice	5
D. Pharmacoepidemiology	10

Finally, the APA (1996) curriculum also includes a practicum designed to be an intensive, closely supervised experience involving exposure to a range of patients and diagnoses. Such a practicum placement would include inpatient and outpatient settings and would expose the practitioner to acute, short-term, and maintenance medication strategies. Ideally, trainees would treat a wide range and sufficient number of patients so they can gain experience with patients representing a mix of age, gender, disability, and ethnicity. To achieve competency in treating a sufficiently diverse patient population, the APA has set a minimum goal of 100 patients for whom the trainee assumes direct clinical responsibility. The patient mix should be relevant to the trainee's current and future practice.

Additional didactic material, such as the sequence in pharmacotherapeutics outlined previously, may be included as seminars or colloquia during clinical training, as should additional training in physical and laboratory assessment. Supervision should be provided by qualified practitioners with demonstrated skills and experience in clinical psychopharmacology (APA, 1996). The APA recommends a minimum of 2 hours of weekly supervision.

LEVELS OF TRAINING

Over the past several years, executive committee members within Division 16, School Psychology, Section 1 on Clinical Child Psychology of Division 12, Clinical Psychology, and the Bureau of Educational Affairs of the APA, made significant efforts to examine systemically the psychopharmacology training needs of psychologists who work with children and adolescents. The consensus of numerous reports is that practicing psychologists desire and need additional training in the area of psychopharmacology (Barkley, Conners, et al., 1990; C. L. Carlson & Kubiszyn, 1994; Piotrowski & Keller, 1996). For this reason, many of the curricula developed are at the postdoctoral level.

There is significant momentum within the APA to study the training needs of psychologists who are the providers of mental health services to children and adolescents. Several task forces systematically explored these issues (Barkley, Conners, et al., 1990; C. L. Carlson & Kubiszyn, 1994). The rationale is that as our understanding of the role of neurobiology in human behavior increases, we have a concomitant need to incorporate biological approaches in managing behavior. Some experts argued that a psychologist who works with a pediatric population must have specific training in pediatric psychopharmacology by means of formal coursework (Balster, 1990; Barkley, Conners, et al., 1990). Further, experts suggest that some of the traditional courses required in the training of clinical and school psychologists, including assessment and consultation, should encompass the study of the appropriate pharmacotherapies for specific childhood disorders as well as the assessment of medication response (Barkley, Conners, et al., 1990).

The APA (Smyer et al., 1992, 1993) identified three levels of preparation in psychopharmacology: (1) basic psychopharmacology education, (2) basic training needs for collaborative practice with physicians (consultation–liaison model), and (3) prescription privileges. Each level presupposes competencies at the previous level. Further, each level represents an increasing responsibility for medication decisions and an exponentially increased requirement pertaining to the amount of prior education, training, and experience. Recognizing the need to improve implementation of combined psychopharmacological and psychosocial treatment, the Center for Mental Health Services of the National Institutes of Health awarded a contract to the APA to develop the first two levels of training.

The first level of training encompasses fundamental knowledge of the biological bases of neuropsychopharmacology, including both the neurobiology of brain function and the means by which various drugs affect the neurotransmitters (Smyer et al., 1992, 1993). This level also includes the mastery of the various agents employed to manage mental disorders. The Level 1 curriculum represents the minimum training necessary for practicing psychologists. The APA recommended that, for clinical, counseling, neuropsychology, and school psychology programs, the Level 1 training include a formal 3- to 5-credit one-semester psychopharmacology course, preceded by a course in the biological bases of behavior. For practicing psychologists who already completed degree requirements, the APA recommended continuing education on the topic.

Level 1

The first level of training includes the following nine modules with related learning objectives and reference material: (1) biological basis of psychopharmacological treatment, (2 and 3) principles of psychopharmacological treatment (two modules are devoted to this topic), (4) clinical psychopharmacology, (5) psychopharmacological treatment of psychoactive substance abuse disorders, (6) psychopharmacological treatment of psychotic disorders, (7) psychopharmacological treatment of mood disorders, (8) psychopharmacological treatment of anxiety disorders, and (9) psychopharmacological treatment of developmental disorders (Kilbey et al., 1995). Each module incorporates summary of purpose, learning objectives, major content areas, sample examination questions, and resources for teaching (e.g., books, articles, and major journals in the field).

Level 1 training in the area of pediatric psychopharmacology is incorporated in the module on developmental disorders, which introduces the psychopharmacological treatment of disorders of development from a life-span perspective. Specifically, the module focuses on the clinical application of pharmacotherapies employed for childhood emotional and behavioral disorders, developmental disabilities believed to have a neuropathological etiology, acquired brain injuries including trauma to the CNS, seizure and tic disorders, organic syndromes arising in midlife or thereafter (e.g., Huntington's and Parkinson's diseases), and, finally, diseases associated with dementia (e.g., Alzheimer's and Pick's diseases).

The module reviews the scope and characteristics of the specific disorders for which pharmacotherapy is likely to prove efficacious and beneficial in the long term. Psychotropic agents commonly employed to treat such disorders are discussed, with a focus on the known or presumed mechanisms of action, special considerations in pharmacokinetics, therapeutic and adverse effects, and the impact of these psychotropic agents on cognition and learning. Finally, ethical and moral considerations are reviewed (Kilbey et al., 1995).

The module assists psychologists in acquiring knowledge of the following topics: (1) childhood disorders for which psychopharmacological treatments are frequently employed; (2) developmental disorders for which psychotropic medications are appropriate and frequently employed; (3) drug classes used in treating children, adolescents, and adults with developmental disabilities, acquired brain injuries, cognitive syndromes, seizure disorders, and diseases associated with dementia; (4) assessment of efficacy and adverse effects of pharmacotherapy in children, adolescents, and adults with cognitive disorders; (5) the role of social and other environmental interventions in drug therapy; and (6) moral and ethical considerations in using pharmacotherapy with minors or individuals affected by cognitive impairments, developmental disabilities, acquired brain injuries, or various dementias.

The major content areas of the module include the following:

   I. Classification of Childhood and Adolescent Psychiatric and Developmental Disorders
   II. Tic and Seizure Disorders
   III. Classification of Disorders of Development
   IV. Acquired Brain Injuries and Cognitive Disorders Arising in Midlife and Later Years
   V. Relation of Social and Other Environmental Interventions to Pharmacotherapy
   VI. Multimodal Therapies
   VII. Classification of Psychotropic Drugs for Special Populations (Children, Adolescents, Adults with Acquired Brain Injuries, and Adults with Developmental Disabilities)
   VIII. Special Considerations in the Assessment of Pharmacotherapy Response and Adverse Effects
   IX. Special Issues Pertaining to Pharmacokinetics in Children, Adolescents, and Adults
   X. Moral and Ethical Issues in the Pharmacotherapy of Children, Adolescents, and Other Special Populations

Level 2

Level 2 training aims to provide the broad knowledge base and skills necessary for psychologists who collaborate with licensed prescribers to manage pharmacotherapy regimens for various psychiatric disorders and integrate such treatments with other psychotherapies and special education programs (Smyer et al., 1992, 1993). Level 2 builds on the introductory Level I curriculum by incorporating more material on specific populations and by including extensive supervised experience with specific populations in managing psychopharmacological treatment. Level 2 training assumes psychologists can play a substantial role in decisions about prescribing medications for children and adolescents.

Level 2 training includes in-depth material about the pharmacology of behaviorally active medication, as well as a comprehensive working of psychodiagnosis, pathophysiology, physical assessment, laboratory tests, drug interactions, developmental psychopharmacology, substance abuse treatment, adverse side effects of various agents, and emergency treatment (Kilbey et al., 1996). It also includes a supervised practicum in which an internship might be modified to include additional experiences in psychopharmacology clinics and provide opportunities to work with physicians to determine whether a particular individual is an appropriate candidate for psychotropic medication. Supervised professional experience can also include attendance at grand rounds in a psychiatric teaching hospital, co-therapy, and emergency treatment experiences, in addition to other supervised clinical experiences.

A prototypical training program at the doctoral level would include two additional didactic courses and a weekly practicum in the specialty area for 1 year (Kilbey et al., 1996). At the internship and postdoctoral residency program level, the supervised experience would include the equivalent of a 4-month rotation in a specialty area with increasing emphasis on supervised professional experience. In continuing professional education programs for licensed practitioners, the program would encompass 8 hours a month of didactic training and 4 hours a week of supervised professional experience in a particular specialty area for 1 year. The modules were developed so that the same material could be acquired longitudinally throughout the sequence of doctoral, internship, and postdoctoral experiences.

The modules in the Level 2 curriculum include the following: (1) child and adolescent populations, (2) populations with mental retardation or developmental disabilities, (3) populations with serious mental illnesses, and (4) geriatric populations. Each module emphasizes pharmacotherapies, pharmacological management of comorbid disorders, treatment settings (e.g., research hospitals, inner-city hospitals, and rural settings), treatment teams, substance abuse, gender, ethnicity, physical disability, sexual orientation, and environment (Kilbey et al., 1996). The program emphasizes specific populations because of their clearly identified needs. The child and adolescent module addresses professional and legal issues, assessment, pharmacological issues, unique aspects of psychopharmacotherapy for youth with developmental and medical conditions, specific treatment issues related to children and adolescents, and research in pediatric psychopharmacology. Future modules may add a psychopharmacological dimension to existing training programs to focus on other populations and problems (e.g., neuropsychology, substance abuse, and rural populations).

Within the professional and legal areas, learning objectives require the acquisition of advanced knowledge and understanding of the collaborative relationship between the psychologist and pediatrician, psychiatrist, and family practitioner (Kilbey et al., 1996). This area addresses benefits and difficulties associated with a collaborative practice that fosters an integrative relationship in the care of children and adolescents. In addition, information is provided about legal and ethical issues central to a collaborative practice (i.e., scope of practice limitations, confidentiality, and informed consent).

The area of assessment emphasizes the assessment and monitoring of physical, behavioral, emotional, and cognitive effects of pharmacotherapies on children, adolescents, and adults with specific developmental or medical disabilities (Kilbey et al., 1996). This part of the module also highlights differences in the way children and adolescents respond to pharmacological agents as compared to adults. The module addresses basic tenets in pharmacology, including pharmacokinetics and mechanisms of drug actions (pharmacodynamics) as they relate to (1) normally developing pediatric populations, (2) pediatric populations with psychiatric disturbances, (3) pediatric populations with developmental and/or physical disabilities requiring medication, and (4) pediatric populations with developmental disabilities with comorbid psychiatric disturbances. Topics include routes of drug administration, distribution, and elimination; pharmacokinetics; tolerance and dependence; and pediatric pharmacokinetics.

The module also addresses some unique issues of youth with developmental and medical conditions, including the interaction between psychopharmacological treatment and developmental/medical conditions that might affect both adverse side effects and treatment outcome (Kilbey et al., 1996). In addition, other special treatment issues in pediatric psychopharmacology relate to social and environmental factors that influence medication administration, efficacy, and adverse side effects. The module emphasizes the role of institutions, including schools, residential treatment facilities, and psychiatric facilities, as they influence pediatric psychopharmacology. Moreover, an understanding of the various phases in psychopharmacotherapy is essential, including the decision to initiate pharmacotherapy, assessment of long-term benefits and adverse side effects, and the consideration to discontinue pharmacotherapy. Practitioners also need to understand the interaction between psychopharmacotherapy and various nonsomatic psychotherapies. An understanding of the efficacy of various psychotropic medications, either in combination with psychotherapy or alone, is important. Finally, practitioners need to know how to assess and manage nonadherence with prescribed psychopharmacotherapy.

Level 3

The third level of training is consistent with the training in other professions that have prescription privileges and that are limited only by scope of practice (i.e., dentists, nurse practitioners, optometrists, and podiatrists) (Smyer et al., 1992, 1993). In accordance with this model, psychologists would be limited to prescribing medications that specifically relate to their scope of practice. Thus, training at Level 3 addresses psychotropic drugs for specific conditions and the idiosyncratic physical, environmental, and mental status that may influence behavioral and physical response to the medication. Should states promulgate statutes granting prescription privileges to psychologists, specialized training programs in psychopharmacology would need to be a core component of graduate programs in applied psychology. Finally, sufficient postdoctoral supervised clinical experiences also are needed. The specific content of this curriculum is currently being developed under the auspices of the Education Directorate of the APA.

RESEARCH ISSUES

Not only will training psychologists in psychopharmacology benefit practitioners who work collaboratively with the physicians who prescribe medication, it also will provide psychologists with greater opportunities in psychopharmacology research (Smyer et al., 1993). Given their scientist–practitioner training, psychologists can bring new discipline and experience to pediatric psychopharmacology. As Smyer et al. (1993) point out, psychologists made important contributions to both basic and clinical psychopharmacology. Increased involvement of psychologists in psychopharmacology will bring new expertise in scientific study that will contribute to advances in our understanding of the use and abuses of various drugs.

These developments require additional faculty with expertise in pediatric psychopharmacology to supervise graduate students in research and mentor other faculty members. Both faculty and students need training in models of drug development, measurement and design strategies, and issues pertaining to safety and abuse liability.

In addition to designing and directing acute trials, long-term follow-up trials, and multimodal trials, researchers can make unique contributions to the literature with studies in such areas as children's development as it mediates response to various psychotropic agents, consumer satisfaction, and cost-effectiveness of pharmacological treatment. Researchers also can contribute to meta-analytic strategies in summarizing the array of research that is already available.

As psychologists become increasingly involved in psychopharmacology research, they will need access to the seminal journals and the capacity to retrieve the most current literature in the field. As Smyer et al. (1993) pointed out, psychologists can take a leadership role in integrating science and practice through developing new psychopharmacology journals specifically designed for psychologists in clinical practice.

The financial resources necessary for conducting psychopharmacology research with children and adolescents must be addressed. Potential funding sources are the National Institute of Mental Health, the National Institute on Drug Abuse, and the Office of Education, as well as pharmaceutical firms and private foundations. The support of various federal agencies for research on the effects of psychotropic medication on learning and behavior will be important in further understanding both the efficacy and safety of various psychotropic medications for children and adolescents. Thus, both federal and private supporters of research should be aware of research in psychopharmacology that is conducted by psychologists (Smyer et al., 1993).

CONCLUSIONS

Psychologists who provide clinical services to children and adolescents will have increasing opportunities to work with youth who are being treated with psychotropic medication. Consequently, psychologists will be asked to consult with other health care providers about decisions to use medication and predict medication response for children and adolescents. These consultation efforts will increase the demands for training psychologists at the predoctoral, postdoctoral, and continuing education levels. Numerous training prototypes are available, and training may be adapted to the level of need. With psychologists' increasing involvement in psychopharmacology comes a concomitant growth of scholarship and research in the field, requiring additional faculty development and providing new employment opportunities for psychologists who are trained in psychopharmacology. Psychologists also will need new venues for dissemination of psychopharmacology research. Identifying sources for funding for laboratory research and clinical trials will be crucial. As psychologists in pediatric psychopharmacology increase their involvement in clinical practice and research, they can build a sound empirical foundation on which to base the clinical use of various behaviorally active medications, leading to improved knowledge of the safety and efficacy of these agents.

Psychologists can serve as important members of the medication treatment team by providing empirical data for designating target behaviors that are apt to be responsive to pharmacotherapy. Psychologists have a spectrum of assessment tools and knowledge of important developmental issues that may mediate children's responses to medication. Thus, these professionals' contributions to the clinical and empirical advances of pediatric psychopharmacology cannot be overestimated. In addition, they play a critical role in the systematic evaluation of the effects of the medication to document any cognitive and/or behavioral toxicities. Psychologists also have important roles in advocating for systematic research that evaluates the clinical efficacy of numerous psychopharmacological agents, many of which receive far too little empirical attention in relation to their widespread clinical use. Finally, psychologists can advocate for studies of the long-term effects of these pharmacotherapies on children and adolescents.

References

♦

Abbott Pharmaceuticals. (1996). *Important drug warning* [Letter]. North Chicago: Author.

Achenbach, T. M. (1991a). *Manual for the Child Behavior Checklist/4–18 and 1991 Profile.* Burlington: University of Vermont, Department of Psychiatry.

Achenbach, T. M. (1991b). *Manual for the Teachers Report Form and 1991 Profile.* Burlington: University of Vermont, Department of Psychiatry.

Achenbach, T. M. (1991c). *Manual for the Youth Self-Report and 1991 Profile.* Burlington: University of Vermont, Department of Psychiatry.

Achenbach, T. M., & Edelbrock, C. (1983). *Manual for the Child Behavior Checklist and Revised Child Behavior Profile.* Burlington: University of Vermont, Department of Psychiatry.

Achenbach, T. M., McConaughy, S. H., & Howell, C. T. (1987). Child/adolescent behavioral and emotional problems: Implications of cross-informant correlations for situational specificity. *Psychological Bulletin, 101,* 213–232.

Adams, K., & Bielauskas, L. A. (1994). Should vs. could: A reply to Salmons. *Journal of Clinical Psychology in Medical Settings, 1,* 209–215.

Akari, M., Takagi, A., Higuchi, I., & Sugita, H. (1988). Neuroleptic malignant syndrome: Caffeine contracture of single muscle fibers and muscle pathology. *Neurology, 38,* 297–301.

Alessi, N., Naylor, M. W., Ghaziuddin, M., & Zubieta, J. K. (1994). Update on lithium carbonate therapy in children and adolescents. *Journal of the American Academy of Child and Adolescent Psychiatry, 33,* 291–304.

Alexandris, A., & Lundell, F. W. (1968). Effect of thioridazine, amphetamine and placebo on the hyperkinetic syndrome and cognitive area in mentally deficient children. *Canadian Medical Association Journal, 98,* 92–96.

Allen, A. J., Leonard, H., & Swedo, S. (1995). Current knowledge of medications for the treatment of childhood anxiety disorders. *Journal of the American Academy of Child and Adolescent Psychiatry, 34,* 976–986.

Aman, M. G. (1978). Drugs, learning, and psychotherapies. In J. S. Werry (Ed.), *Pediatric psychopharmacology: The use of behavior modifying drugs in children* (pp. 79–108). New York: Brunner/Mazel.

187

Aman, M. G. (1980). Psychotropic drugs and learning problems—A selective review. *Journal of Learning Disabilities, 13,* 87–97.

Aman, M. G. (1984). Drugs and learning in mentally retarded persons. In G. D. Burrows & J. S. Werry (Eds.), *Advances in human psychopharmacology* (Vol. 3, pp. 121–163). Greenwich, CT: JAI Press.

Aman, M. G. (1993). Monitoring and measuring drug effects: II. Behavioral, emotional, and cognitive effects. In J. S. Werry & M. G. Aman (Eds.), *Practitioner's guide to psychoactive drugs for children and adolescents* (pp. 99–159). New York: Plenum.

Aman, M. G., Field, C. J., & Bridgman, G. D. (1985). City-wide survey of drug patterns among noninstitutionalized retarded persons. *Applied Research in Mental Retardation, 6,* 159–171.

Aman, M. G., & Singh, N. N. (1988). *Psychopharmacotherapy of the developmental disabilities.* Berlin: Springer-Verlag.

Aman, M. G., & Singh, N. N. (1991). Pharmacological intervention. In J. L. Matson & J. A. Mulick (Eds.), *Handbook of mental retardation* (2nd ed., pp. 347–372). New York: Pergamon Press.

Aman, M. G., & Werry, J. S. (1982). Methylphenidate and diazepam in severe reading retardation. *Journal of the American Academy of Child and Adolescent Psychiatry, 21,* 31–37.

Aman, M. G., Werry, J. S., Paxton, J. W., & Turbott, S. H. (1987). Effect of sodium valproate on psychomotor performance in children as a function of dose, fluctuations in concentration, and diagnosis. *Epilepsia, 28,* 115–124.

Aman, M. G., Werry, J. S., Paxton, J. W., Turbott, S. H., & Stewart, A. W. (1990). Effects of carbamazepine on psychomotor performance in children as a function of drug concentration, seizure type, and time of medication. *Epilepsia, 31,* 51–60.

Aman, M. G., & Wolford, P. L. (1995). Consumer satisfaction with involvement in drug research: A social validity study. *Journal of the American Academy of Child and Adolescent Psychiatry, 34,* 940–945.

Ambrosini, P. J., Bianchi, M. D., Rabinovich, H., & Elia, J. (1993). Antidepressant treatments in children and adolescents: I. Affective disorders. *Journal of the American Academy of Child and Adolescent Psychiatry, 32,* 1–6.

Ambrosini, P. J., Bianchi, M. D., Rabinovich, H., & Elia, J. (1993b). Antidepressant treatments in children and adolescents II. Anxiety, physical, and behavioral disorders. *Journal of the American Academy of Child and Adolescent Psychiatry, 32,* 483–493.

Ambrosini, P. J., Metz, C., Prabucki, K., & Lee, J. (1989). Videotape reliability of the third revised edition of the K-SADS. *Journal of the American Academy of Child and Adolescent Psychiatry, 28,* 723–728.

American Academy of Pediatrics. (1985). Behavioral and cognitive effects of anticonvulsant therapy. *Pediatrics, 76,* 644–647.

American Psychiatric Association. (1987). *Diagnostic and statistical manual of mental disorders* (3rd ed., rev.). Washington, DC: Author.

American Psychiatric Association. (1994). *Diagnostic and statistical manual of mental disorders* (4th ed.) Washington, DC: Author.

American Psychological Association. (1996, February). *Recommended postdoctoral training in psychopharmacology for prescription privileges: Interim document approved by council.* Washington, DC: Author.

Amirkhan, J. (1982). Expectancies and attributions for hyperactive and medicated hyperactive students. *Journal of Abnormal Child Psychology, 10,* 265–276.

Anderson, L. T., Campbell, M., Adams, P., Small, A. M., Perry, R., & Shell, J. (1989). The effects of haloperidol on discrimination learning and behavioral symptoms in autistic children. *Journal of Autism and Developmental Disorders, 19,* 227–239.

Anderson, L. T., Campbell, M., Grega, D. M., Perry, R., Small, A. M., & Green, W. H. (1984). Haloperidol in the treatment of infantile autism: Effects on learning and behavioral symptoms. *American Journal of Psychiatry, 141,* 1195–1202.

Apter, A., Ratzone, G., King, R. A., Weizman, A., Iancu, I., Binder, M., & Riddle, M. A. (1994). Fluvoxamine open-label treatment of adolescent inpatients with obsessive–compulsive disorder or depression. *Journal of the American Academy of Child and Adolescent Psychiatry, 33,* 342–348.

Atkins, M. S., & Pelham, W. E. (1991). School-based assessment of attention deficit-hyperactivity disorder. *Journal of Learning Disabilities, 24,* 197–204.

Ax, R. K., & Babcock, D. J. (1995). *A basic course in psychopharmacology for predoctoral psychology interns: Training manual.* Washington, DC: Federal Bureau of Prisons.

Ayd, F. J. (1995). *Lexicon of psychiatry, neurology, and the neurosciences.* Baltimore: Williams & Wilkins.

Balster, R. L. (1990). Predoctoral psychopharmacology training for clinical/counseling psychologists. *Psychopharmacology Newsletter, 23,* 3–4.

Balthazor, M. J., Wagner, R. K., & Pelham, W. E. (1991). The specificity of the effects of stimulant medication on classroom learning-related measures of cognitive processing for attention deficit disorder children. *Journal of Abnormal Child Psychology, 19,* 35–92.

Bangs, M. E., Petti, T. A., & Mark-David, J. (1994). Fluoxetine-induced memory impairment in an adolescent. *Journal of the American Academy of Child and Adolescent Psychiatry, 33,* 1303–1306.

Barkley, R. A. (1977). A review of stimulant drug research with hyperactive children. *Journal of Child Psychology and Psychiatry, 18,* 137–165.

Barkley, R. A. (1988). Child behavior rating scales and checklists. In M. Rutter, A. H. Tuma, & I. S. Lann (Eds.), *Assessment and diagnosis in child psychopathology* (pp. 113–155).New York: Guilford Press.

Barkley, R. A. (1990). *Attention-deficit/hyperactivity disorder: A handbook for diagnosis and treatment.* New York: Guilford Press.

Barkley, R. A. (1991). The ecological validity of laboratory and analogue assessment methods of ADHD symptoms. *Journal of Abnormal Child Psychology, 19,* 149–178.

Barkley, R. A., Conners, C. K., Barclay, A., Gadow, K., Gittelman, R., Sprague, R. L., & Swanson, J. (1990). Task force report: The appropriate role of clinical child psychologists in the prescribing of psychoactive medication for children. *Journal of Clinical Child Psychology, 19*(Suppl.), 1–38.

Barkley, R. A., & Cunningham, C. E. (1979). The effects of methylphenidate on the mother–child interactions of hyperactive children. *Archives of General Psychiatry, 36,* 201–208.

Barkley, R. A., DuPaul, G. J., & Costello, A. J. (1993). Stimulants. In J. S. Werry & M. G. Aman (Eds.), *Practitioner's guide to psychoactive drugs for children and adolescents* (pp. 205–237). New York: Plenum.

Barkley, R. A., Fischer, M., Newby, R. F., & Breen, M. J. (1988). Development of a multimethod clinical protocol for assessing stimulant drug responses in children with attention deficit disorder. *Journal of Clinical Child Psychology, 17,* 14–24.

Barkley, R. A., & Grodzinsky, G. M. (1994). Are tests of frontal lobe functions used in the diagnosis of attention deficit disorders? *The Clinical Neuropsychologist, 8,* 121–139.

Barkley, R. A., Grodzinsky, G., & DuPaul, G. J. (1992). Frontal lobe functions in attention deficit disorder with and without hyperactivity: A review and research report. *Journal of Abnormal Child Psychology, 20,* 163–168.

Barkley, R. A., Karlsson, J., Strzelecki, E., & Murphy, J. V. (1984). Effects of age and Ritalin dosage on the mother–child interactions of hyperactive children. *Journal of Consulting and Clinical Psychology, 52,* 750–758.

Barkley, R. A., McMurray, M. B., Edelbrock, C. S., & Robbins, K. (1990). Side effects of methylphenidate in children with attention deficit hyperactivity disorder: A systematic, placebo-controlled evaluation. *Pediatrics, 86,* 184–192.

Barrickman, L., Noyes, R., Kuperman, S., Schumacher, E., & Verda, M. (1991). Treatment of ADHD with fluoxetine: A preliminary trial. *Journal of the American Academy of Child and Adolescent Psychiatry, 30,* 762–767.

Barrickman, L., Perry, P. J., Allen, A. J., Kuperman, S., Arndt, S. V., Herrmann, K. J., & Schumacher, E. (1995). Bupropion versus methylphenidate in the treatment of attention-deficit hyperactivity disorder. *Journal of the American Academy of Child and Adolescent Psychiatry, 34,* 649–657.

Beery, S. H., Quay, H. C., & Pelham, W. E. (1995, August). *Behavioral disinhibition and response to methylphenidate in children with attention deficit hyperactivity disorder.* Paper presented at the annual meeting of the American Psychological Association, New York.

Berg, C. J., Rapoport, J. L., & Flament, M. (1986). The Leyton Obsessional Inventory—Child Version. *Journal of the American Academy of Child Psychiatry, 25,* 84–91.

Berg, I., Butler, A., Ellis, M., & Foster, J. (1993). Psychiatric aspects of epilepsy in childhood treated with carbamazepine, phenytoin, or sodium valproate: A random trial. *Developmental Medicine and Child Neurology, 35,* 149–157.

Bernstein, G. A., Garfinkel, B. D., & Borchardt, C. M. (1990). Comparative studies of pharmacotherapy for school refusal. *Journal of the American Academy of Child and Adolescent Psychiatry, 29,* 773–781.

Biederman, J. (1987). Clonazepam in the treatment of prepubertal children with panic-like symptoms. *Journal of Clinical Psychiatry, 48,* 38–41.

Biederman, J., Baldessarini, R. J., Wright, V., Keenan, K., & Faraone, S. (1993). A double-blind placebo controlled study of desipramine in the treatment of ADD: III. Lack of impact of comorbidity and family history factors on clinical response. *Journal of the American Academy of Child and Adolescent Psychiatry, 32,* 199–204.

Biederman, J., Baldessarini, R. J., Wright, V., Knee, D., & Harmatz, J. S. (1989). A double-blind placebo controlled study of desipramine in the treatment of ADD: I. Efficacy. *Journal of the American Academy of Child and Adolescent Psychiatry, 28,* 777–784.

Birmaher, B., Baker, R., Kapur, S., Quintana, H., & Ganguli, R. (1992). Clozapine for the treatment of adolescents with schizophrenia. *Journal of the American Academy of Child and Adolescent Psychiatry, 31,* 160–164.

Birmaher, B., Waterman, G. S., Ryan, N., Cully, M., Balach, L., Ingram, J., & Brodsky, M. (1994). Fluoxetine for childhood anxiety disorders. *Journal of the American Academy of Child and Adolescent Psychiatry, 33,* 993–999.

Black, B., & Uhde, T.W. (1994). Treatment of elective mutism with fluoxetine: A double-blind, placebo-controlled study. *Journal of the American Academy of Child and Adolescent Psychiatry, 33,* 1000–1006.

Blackwell, B., & Currah, J. (1973). The psychopharmacology of nocturnal enuresis. In I. Kolvin, R. C. McKeith, & S. R. Meadows (Eds.), *Bladder control and enuresis* (pp. 231–257). London: Heinemann.

Blouin, A. G., Bornstein, R. A., & Trites, R. L. (1978). Teenage alcohol use among hyperactive and nonhyperactive children: A five-year follow-up study. *Journal of Pediatric Psychology, 3,* 188–194.

Borden, K. A., & Brown, R. T. (1989). Attributional outcomes: The subtle messages of treatment for attention deficit disorder. *Cognitive Therapy and Research, 13,* 147–160.

Boulos, C., Kutcher, S., Gardner, D., & Young, E. (1992). An open-naturalistic trial of fluoxetine in adolescents and young adults with treatment-resistant major depression. *Journal of Child and Adolescent Psychopharmacology, 2,* 103–111.

Bowen, J., Fenton, T., & Rappaport, L. (1991). Stimulant medication and attention deficit-hyperactivity disorder: The child's perspective. *American Journal of Diseases of Children, 145,* 291–295.

Bradley, C. (1937). The behavior of children receiving benzedrine. *American Journal of Psychiatry, 94,* 577–585.

Brent, D. A., Crumrine, P. K., Varma, R. R., Allan, M., & Allman, C. (1987). Phenobarbital treatment and major depressive disorder in children with epilepsy. *Pediatrics, 80,* 909–917.

Breuning, S. E. (1983). Effects of thioridazine on the intellectual performance of mentally retarded drug responders and nonresponders. *Archives of General Psychiatry, 40,* 309–313.

Briant, R. H. (1978). An introduction to clinical pharmacology. In J. S. Werry (Ed.), *Pediatric psychopharmacology: The use of behavior modifying drugs in children* (pp. 3–28). New York: Brunner/Mazel.

Brown, J. L., & Bing, S. R. (1976). Drugging children: Child abuse by professionals. In G. P. Koocher (Ed.), *Children's rights and the mental health professions* (pp. 219–228). New York: Wiley.

Brown, R. T., & Borden, K. A. (1989). Neuropsychological effects of stimulant medication on children's learning and behavior. In C. R. Reynolds & E.

Fletcher-Janzen (Eds.), *Handbook of clinical child neuropsychology* (pp. 443–474). New York: Plenum.

Brown, R. T., Borden, K. A., Wynne, M. E., Clingerman, S. R., & Spunt, A. L. (1987). Compliance with pharmacological and cognitive treatments for attention deficit disorder. *Journal of the American Academy of Child and Adolescent Psychiatry, 26,* 521–526.

Brown, R. T., Borden, K. A., Wynne, M. E., Schleser, R., & Clingerman, S. R. (1986). Methylphenidate and cognitive therapy with ADD children: A methodological reconsideration. *Journal of Abnormal Psychology, 14,* 481–497.

Brown, R. T., & Dingle, A. (1994). Overview of psychopharmacology in children and adolescents. *School Psychology Quarterly, 9,* 4–25.

Brown, R. T., Dingle, A. D., & Dreelin, E. (1997). Neuropsychological effects of stimulant medication on children's learning and behavior. In C. R. Reynolds & E. Fletcher-Janzen (Eds.), *Handbook of clinical child neuropsychology* (2nd ed., pp. 539–572). New York: Wiley.

Brown, R. T., Dingle, A. D., & Landau, S. (1994). Overview of psychopharmacology in children and adolescents. *School Psychology Quarterly, 9,* 5–30.

Brown, R. T., & Donegan, J. E. (1995). The growing impact of neurology. In D. K. Reid, W. P. Hresko, & H. L. Swanson (Eds.), *Cognitive approaches to learning disabilities* (3rd ed., pp. 153–211). Austin, TX: Pro-Ed.

Brown, R. T., Jaffe, S. L., Magee, H., & Silverstein, J. (1992). Methylphenidate and adolescents hospitalized with conduct disorder: Dose effects on classroom behavior, academic performance, and impulsivity. *Journal of Clinical Child Psychology, 20,* 282–292.

Brown, R. T., Jaffe, S., Silverstein, J., & McGee, H. (1991). Methylphenidate and adolescents hospitalized with conduct disorder: Dose effects on classroom behavior, academic performance, and impulsivity. *Journal of Clinical Child Psychology, 20,* 282–292.

Brown, R. T., Lee, D. O., & Donegan, J. E. (in press). Psychopharmacotherapy with school-aged children. In C. R. Reynolds & T. Gutkin (Eds.), *Handbook of school psychology* (3rd ed.). New York: Wiley.

Brown, R. T., & Morris, M. K. (1994). Central nervous system. In V. S. Ramachandran (Ed.), *Encyclopedia of human behavior* (Vol. 1, pp. 537–547). San Diego, CA: Academic Press.

Brown, R. T., & Quay, L. C. (1977). Reflection-impulsivity in normal and behavior disordered boys. *Journal of Abnormal Child Psychology, 5,* 457–462.

Brown, R. T., & Sexson, S. B. (1988). A controlled trial of methylphenidate in black adolescents: Attentional, behavioral, and physiological effects. *Clinical Pediatrics, 27,* 74–81.

Brown, R. T., & Sexson, S. B. (1989). Effects of methylphenidate on cardiovascular responses in attention deficit hyperactivity disordered adolescents. *Journal of Adolescent Health Care, 10,* 179–183.

Brown, R. T., & Sleator, E. K. (1979). Methylphenidate in hyperkinetic children: Differences in dose effects on impulsive behavior. *Pediatrics, 64,* 408–411.

Brown, R. T., Wynne, M. E., & Medenis, R. (1985). Methylphenidate and cognitive therapy: A comparison of treatment approaches with hyperactive boys. *Journal of Abnormal Child Psychology, 13,* 69–87.

Buhrmester, D., Whalen, C. K., MacDonald, V., Henker, B., & Hinshaw, S. P. (1992). Prosocial behavior in hyperactive boys: Effects of stimulant medication and comparison with normal boys. *Journal of Abnormal Child Psychology, 20,* 103–121.

Buitelaar, J. K., Van der Gaag, R. J., Swaab-Barneveld, H., & Kuiper, M. (1995). Prediction of clinical response to methylphenidate in children with attention-deficit/hyperactivity disorder. *Journal of the American Academy of Child and Adolescent Psychiatry, 34,* 1025–1032.

Bukstein, O. (1992). Overview of pharmacological treatment. In V. B. Van Hasselt & M. Hersen (Eds.), *Handbook of behavior therapy and pharmacotherapy for children* (pp. 213–232). Boston: Allyn & Bacon.

Burns, S. M., DeLeon, P. H., Chemtob, C. M., & Welch, B. L. (in press). Psychotropic medication: A new technique for psychology? *Psychotherapy: Theory, Research, Practice, and Training.*

Cade, J. F. J. (1949). Lithium salts for the treatment of psychotic excitement. *Medical Journal of Australia, 2,* 349–352.

Caine, E. D., Ludlow, C. L., Polinsky, R. J., & Ebert, M. H. (1984). Provocative drug testing in Tourette's syndrome: *d*- and *l*-amphetamine and haloperidol. *Journal of the American Academy of Child and Adolescent Psychiatry, 23,* 147–152.

Cameron, O. G., & Thyer, B. A. (1985). Treatment of pavor nocturnus with alprazolam. *Journal of Clinical Psychiatry, 46,* 504.

Camfield, C. S., Chaplin, S., Doyle, A. B., Shapiro, S. H., Cummings, C., & Camfield, P. R. (1979). Side effects of phenobarbital in toddlers: Behavioral and cognitive aspects. *Journal of Pediatrics, 95,* 361–365.

Campbell, G. A., Small, A. M., Green, W. H., Jennings, S. J., Perry, R., Bennett, W. G., & Anderson, L. (1984). Behavioral efficacy of haloperidol and lithium carbonate: A comparison in hospitalized aggressive children with conduct disorder. *Archives of General Psychiatry, 41,* 650–656.

Campbell, M. (1985). Protocol for rating drug-related AIMS, stereotypies, and CPRS assessments. *Psychopharmacology Bulletin, 21,* 1081.

Campbell, M., Adams, P., Perry, R., Spencer, E. K., & Overall, J. E. (1988). Tardive and withdrawal dyskinesia in autistic children: A prospective study. *Psychopharmacology Bulletin, 24,* 251–255.

Campbell, M., Anderson, L. T., Meier, M., Cohen, I. L., Small, A. M., Samit, C., & Sachar, E. J. (1978). A comparison of haloperidol, behavior therapy and their interaction in autistic children. *Journal of the American Academy of Child and Adolescent Psychiatry, 17,* 640–655.

Campbell, M., Cohen, I. L., Perry, R., & Small, A. M. (1989). Psychopharmacological treatment. In T. H. Ollendick & M. Hersen (Eds.), *Handbook of child psychopathology* (2nd ed., pp. 473–497). New York: Plenum.

Campbell, M., Cohen, I. L., & Small, A. M. (1982). Drugs in aggressive behavior. *Journal of the American Academy of Child and Adolescent Psychiatry, 21,* 107–117.

Campbell, M., & Cueva, J. E. (1995a). Psychopharmacology in child and adolescent psychiatry: A review of the past seven years. Part I. *Journal of the American Academy of Child and Adolescent Psychiatry, 34,* 1124–1132.

Campbell, M., & Cueva, J. E. (1995b). Psychopharmacology in child and adolescent psychiatry: A review of the past seven years. Part II. *Journal of the American Academy of Child and Adolescent Psychiatry, 34*, 1262–1272.

Campbell, M., Fish, B., Korein, J., Shapiro, T., Collins, P., & Koh, C. (1972). Lithium and chlorpromazine: A controlled crossover study of hyperactive severely disturbed young children. *Journal of Autism and Child Schizophrenia, 2*, 234–263.

Campbell, M., Gonzalez, N. M., & Silva, R. R. (1992). The pharmacologic treatment of conduct disorders and rage outbursts. In D. Shaffer (Ed.), *The psychiatric clinics of North America* (Vol. 15, pp. 69–85). Philadelphia: Saunders.

Campbell, M., Gonzalez, N. M., Ernst, M., Silva, R. R., & Werry, J. S. (1993). Antipsychotics (neuroleptics). In J. S. Werry & M. G. Aman (Eds.), *Practitioner's guide to psychoactive drugs for children and adolescents* (pp. 269–296). New York: Plenum.

Campbell, M., Green, W. H., & Deutsch, S. I. (1985). *Child and adolescent psychopharmacology.* Beverly Hills, CA: Sage.

Campbell, M., Kafantaris, V., & Cueva, J. E. (1995). An update on the use of lithium carbonate in aggressive children and adolescents with conduct disorder. *Psychopharmacology Bulletin, 31*, 93–102.

Campbell, M., & Malone, R. P. (1991). Mental retardation and psychiatry disorders. *Hospital and Community Psychiatry, 42*, 374–379.

Campbell, M., Overall, J. E., Small, A. M., Sokol, M. S., Spencer, E. K., Adams, P., Foltz, R. L, Monti, K. M., Perry, R., Nobler, M., & Roberts, E. (1989). Naltrexone in autistic children: An acute open dose range tolerance trial. *Journal of the American Academy of Child and Adolescent Psychiatry, 28*, 200–206.

Campbell, M., & Palij, M. (1985). Measurement of side effects including tardive dyskinesia. *Psychopharmacology Bulletin, 21*, 1063–1066.

Campbell, M., Perry, R., & Green, W. H. (1984). The use of lithium in children and adolescents. *Psychosomatics, 25*, 95–106.

Campbell, M., Schulman, D., & Rapoport, J. (1978). The current status of lithium therapy in child and adolescent psychiatry. *Journal of the American Academy of Child and Adolescent Psychiatry, 14*, 717–729.

Campbell, M., Small, A. M., Green, W. H., Jennings, S. J., Perry, R., Bennett, W. G., & Anderson, L. (1984). Behavioral efficacy of haloperidol and lithium carbonate. A comparison in hospitalized aggressive children with conduct disorder. *Archives of General Psychiatry, 41*, 650–656.

Carlson, C. L., & Kubiszyn, T. (1994). Prescription privileges: Psychopharmacology and school psychology: An overview. *School Psychology Quarterly, 9*, 1–3.

Carlson, C. L., Paavola, J., & Talley, R. (1995). Historical, current, and future models of schools as health care delivery settings. *School Psychology Quarterly, 10*, 184–202.

Carlson, C. L., Pelham, W. E., Milich, R., & Dixon, J. (1992). Single and combined effects of methylphenidate and behavior therapy on the classroom performance of children with attention-deficit hyperactivity disorder. *Journal of Abnormal Child Psychology, 20*, 213–232.

Carlson, C. L., Pelham, W. E., Milich, R., & Hoza, B. (1993). ADHD boys' performance and attributions following success and failure: Drug effects and individual differences. *Cognitive Therapy and Research, 17*, 269–287.

Carlson, G. A., Rapport, M. D., Kelly, K. L., & Pataki, C. S. (1992). The effects of methylphenidate and lithium on attention and activity level. *Journal of the American Academy of Child and Adolescent Psychiatry, 31,* 262–270.

Carlson, G. A., Rapport, M. D., Pataki, C. S. & Kelly, K. L. (1992). Lithium in hospitalized children at 4 and 8 weeks: Mood, behavior and cognitive effects. *Journal of Child Psychology and Psychiatry, 33,* 411–425.

Carpenter, R. O., & Vining, E. P. G. (1993). Antiepileptics (anticonvulsants). In J. S. Werry & M. G. Aman (Eds.), *Practitioner's guide to psychoactive drugs for children and adolescents* (pp. 321–346). New York: Plenum.

Castellanos, F. X., & Rapoport, J. L. (1992). Etiology of attention-deficit hyperactivity disorder. *Child and Adolescent Psychiatric Clinics of North America, 2,* 373–384.

Chambers, W. J., Puig-Antich, J., Hirsch, M., Paez, P., Ambrosini, P. J., Tabrizi, M. A. (1985). The assessment of affective disorders in children and adolescents by semistructured interview: Test–retest reliability of the Schedule for Affective Disorders and Schizophrenia for school aged children, present episode version. *Archives of General Psychiatry, 42,* 696–702.

Charles, L., & Schain, R. (1981). A four-year follow-up study of the effects of methylphenidate on the behavior and achievement of hyperactive children. *Journal of Abnormal Child Psychology, 9,* 495–505.

Clay, T. H., Gualtieri, C. T., Evans, R. W., & Gullion, C. M. (1988). Clinical and neuropsychological effects of the novel antidepressant bupropion. *Psychopharmacology Bulletin, 24,* 143–148.

Coffey, B. J. (1990). Anxiolytics for children and adolescents: Traditional and new drugs. *Journal of Child and Adolescent Psychopharmacology, 1,* 57–86.

Cohen, D. J., & Leckman, J. F. (1989). Commentary. *Journal of the American Academy of Child and Adolescent Psychiatry, 28,* 580–582.

Cohen, N. J., & Thompson, L. (1982). Perceptions and attitudes of hyperactive children and their mothers regarding treatment with methylphenidate. *Canadian Journal of Psychiatry, 27,* 40–42.

Como, P. G., & Kurlan, R. (1991). An open label trial of fluoxetine for obsessive compulsive behavior in Gilles de la Tourette's syndrome. *Neurology, 41,* 872–874.

Conners, C. K. (1969). A teacher rating scale for use in drug studies with children. *American Journal of Psychiatry, 126,* 884–888.

Conners, C. K. (1970). Symptom patterns in hyperkinetic neurotic and normal children. *Child Development, 41,* 667–682.

Conners, C. K., & Barkley, R. A. (1985). Rating scales and checklists for child psychopharmacology. *Psychopharmacology Bulletin, 21,* 809–851.

Conners, C. K., & Kronsberg, S. (1985). Measuring activity level in children. *Psychopharmacology Bulletin, 21,* 893–897.

Cook, E. H., Rowlett, R., Jaselskis, C., & Leventhal, B. L. (1992). Fluoxetine treatment of children and adults with autistic disorder and mental retardation. *Journal of the American Academy of Child and Adolescent Psychiatry, 31,* 739–745.

Cross-Calvert, S., & Johnston, C. (1990). Acceptability of treatments for child behavior problems: Issues and implications for future research. *Journal of Clinical Child Psychology, 19,* 61–74.

Cullinan, D., Gadow, K. D., & Epstein, M. H. (1987). Psychotropic drug treatment among learning disabled, mentally retarded, and seriously emotionally disturbed students. *Journal of Abnormal Child Psychology, 15,* 469–477.

Cunningham, C. E., & Barkley, R. A. (1979). The interactions of hyperactive and normal children with their mothers in free play and structured tasks. *Child Development, 50,* 217–224.

Cunningham, M. A., Pillai, V., & Rogers, W. J. B. (1968). Haloperidol in the treatment of children with severe behavioural disorders. *British Journal of Psychiatry, 114,* 845–854.

D'Amato, G. (1962). Chlordiazepoxide in management of school phobia. *Diseases of the Nervous System, 23,* 292–295.

Dager, S. R., & Herich, A. J. (1990). A case of bupropion-associated delirium. *Journal of Clinical Psychiatry, 51,* 307–308.

Dalby, J. T., Kinsbourne, M., & Swanson, J. M. (1989). Self-paced learning in children with attention deficit disorder with hyperactivity. *Journal of Abnormal Child Psychology, 17,* 269–275.

DeLeon, P. H., Folen, R. A., Jennings, F. L., Willis, D. J., & Wright, R. H. (1991). The case for prescription privileges: A logical evolution of professional practice. *Journal of Clinical Child Psychology, 20,* 254–267.

DeLeon, P. H., Fox, R. E., & Graham, S. R. (1991). Prescription privileges: Psychology's next frontier. *American Psychologist, 46,* 384–393.

DeLeon, P. H., Sammons, M. T., & Sexton, J. L. (1995). Focusing on society's real needs: Responsibility and prescription privileges? *American Psychologist, 50,* 1022–1032.

DeLong, G. R., & Aldershof, A. L. (1987). Long-term experience with lithium treatment in childhood: Correlation with clinical diagnosis. *Journal of the American Academy of Child and Adolescent Psychiatry, 26,* 389–394.

DeMers, S. T. (1995). Emerging perspectives on the role of psychologists in the delivery of health and mental health services in schools. *School Psychology Quarterly, 10,* 179–183.

DeVane, C. L., & Sallee, F. R. (1996). Selective serotonin reuptake inhibitors in child and adolescent psychopharmacology: A review of published experience. *Journal of Clinical Psychiatry, 57,* 55–66.

DeVeaugh-Geiss, J., Moroz, G., Biederman, J., Cantwell, D., Fontaine, R., Greist, J.H., Reichler, R., Katz, R., & Landau, P. (1992). Clomipramine in child and adolescent obsessive–compulsive disorder: A multicenter trial. *Journal of the American Academy of Child and Adolescent Psychiatry, 31,* 45–49.

Deykin, E. Y., & MacMahon, B. (1979). The incidence of seizures among children with autistic symptoms. *American Journal of Psychiatry, 126,* 1310–1312.

Dodrill, C. B., & Temkin, N. R. (1989). Motor speed is a contaminating factor in evaluating the "cognitive" effects of phenytoin. *Epilepsia, 30,* 453–457.

Douglas, V. I., Barr, R. G., Amin, K., O'Neill, M. E., & Britton, B. G. (1988). Dosage effects and individual responsivity to methylphenidate in attention deficit disorder. *Journal of Child Psychology and Psychiatry, 29,* 453–475.

Douglas, V. I., Barr, R., Desilets, J., & Sherman, E. (1995). Do high doses of stimulants impair flexible thinking in ADHD? *Journal of the American Academy of Child and Adolescent Psychiatry, 34,* 877–885.

Douglas, V. I., Barr, R. G., O'Neill, M. E., Britton, B. G. (1986). Short-term effects of methylphenidate on the cognitive, learning and academic performance of children with attention deficit disorder in the laboratory and the classroom. *Journal of Child Psychology and Psychiatry, 27,* 191–211.

Douglas, V. I., & Peters, K. (1979). Toward a clearer definition of the attention deficit hyperactive children. In G. A. Hale & M. Lewis (Eds.), *Attentional and cognitive development* (pp. 173–247). New York: Plenum.

DuPaul, G. J., Anastopoulos, A. D., Shelton, T. L., Guevremont, D. C., & Metevia, L. (1992). Multimethod assessment of attention-deficit hyperactivity disorder: The diagnostic utility of clinic-based tests. *Journal of Clinical Child Psychology, 21,* 394–402.

DuPaul, G. J., & Barkley, R. A. (1990). Medication therapy. In R. A. Barkley, *Attention-deficit hyperactivity disorder: A handbook for diagnosis and treatment* (pp. 573–612). New York: Guilford Press.

DuPaul, G. J., Barkley, R. A., & McMurray, M. B. (1994). Response of children with ADHD to methylphenidate: Interaction with internalizing symptoms. *Journal of the American Academy of Child and Adolescent Psychiatry, 33,* 894–903.

DuPaul, G. J., & Kyle, K. E. (1995). Pediatric pharmacology and psychopharmacology. In M. C. Roberts (Ed.), *Handbook of pediatric psychology* (2nd ed., pp. 741–758). New York: Guilford.

DuPaul, G. J., & Rapport, M. (1993). Does methylphenidate normalize the classroom performance of children with attention deficit disorder? *Journal of the American Academy of Child and Adolescent Psychiatry, 32,* 190–198.

Dweck, C. S., & Leggett, E. L. (1988). A social-cognitive approach to motivation and personality. *Psychological Review, 95,* 256–273.

Edelbrock, C. (1978). *Child Attention Problems Scale.* Unpublished manuscript, Pennsylvania State University, University Park, PA.

Elia, J., Welsh, P. A., Gullotta, C. S., & Rapoport, J. L. (1993). Classroom academic performance: Improvement with both methylphenidate and dextroamphetamine in ADHD boys. *Journal of Child Psychology and Psychiatry, 34,* 785–804.

Elliott, S. N. (1988). Acceptability of behavioral treatments in educational settings. In J. C. Witt, S. N. Elliott, & F. M. Gresham (Eds.), *Handbook of behavior therapy in education* (pp. 121–150). New York: Plenum.

Emerson, R., D'Souza, B. J., Vining, E. P., Holden, K. R., Mellits, E. D., & Freeman, J. M. (1981). Stopping medication in children with epilepsy. *New England Journal of Medicine, 304,* 1125–1129.

Engelhardt, D. M., Polizos, P., Waizer, J., & Hoffman, S. P. (1973). A double-blind comparison of fluphenazine and haloperidol in outpatient schizophrenic children. *Journal of Autism and Childhood Schizophrenia, 3,* 128–137.

Epstein, M. H., Matson, J. L., Repp, A., & Helsel, W. J. (1986). Acceptability of treatment alternative as a function of teacher status and student level. *School Psychology Review, 15,* 84–90.

Epstein, M. H., Singh, N. N., Luebke, J., & Stout, C. E. (1991). Psychopharmacological intervention. II. Teacher perceptions of psychotropic medication for students with learning disabilities. *Journal of Learning Disabilities, 24,* 477–483.

Evans, R. W., Clay, T. H., & Gualtieri, C. T. (1987). Carbamazepine in pediatric psychiatry. *Journal of the American Academy of Child and Adolescent Psychiatry, 26,* 2–8.

Evans, R. W., Gualtieri, C. T., & Amara, I. (1986). Methylphenidate and memory: Dissociated effects in hyperactive children. *Psychopharmacology, 90,* 211–216.

Eyberg, S. M., Boggs, S. T., & Algina, J. (1995). New developments in psychosocial, pharmacological, and combined treatments of conduct disorders in aggressive children. *Psychopharmacology Bulletin, 31,* 83–91.

Fang, J. C., Hinrichs, J. V., & Ghoneim, M. M. (1987). Diazepam and memory: Evidence for spared memory function. *Pharmacology, Biochemistry, and Behavior, 28,* 347–352.

Farwell, J. R., Lee, Y. J., Hirtz, D. G., Sulzbacher, S. I., Ellenberg, J. H., & Nelson, K. B. (1990). Phenobarbital for febrile seizures: Effects on intelligence and on seizure recurrence. *New England Journal of Medicine, 322,* 364–369.

Fava, M., Herzog, D. B., Hamburg, P., Reiss, H., Anfang, S., & Rosenbaum, J. F. (1990, April). *A retrospective study of long-term use of fluoxetine in bulimia nervosa.* Paper presented at the Fourth International Conference on Eating Disorders, New York.

Feinberg, M., & Carroll, B. J. (1979). Effects of dopamine agonists in Tourette's disease. *Archives of General Psychiatry, 44,* 1025–1026.

Feldman, S., Denhoff, E., & Denhoff. (1979). The attention disorders and related syndromes: Outcome in adolescence and young adult life. In L. Starr & E. Denhoff (Eds.), *Minimal brain dysfunction: A developmental approach* (pp. 133–148). New York: Mason.

Firestone, P. (1982). Factors associated with children's adherence to stimulant medication. *American Journal of Orthopsychiatry, 52,* 447–457.

Fish, B. (1970). Psychopharmacologic response of chronic schizophrenic adults as predictors of responses in young schizophrenic children. *Psychopharmacology Bulletin 6,* 12–15.

Fisher, R.L., & Fisher, S. (1996). Antidepressants for children: Is scientific support necessary? *Journal of Nervous and Mental Disease, 184,* 99–102.

Fisher, W., Kerbeshian, J., & Burd, L. (1986). A treatable language disorder: Pharmacological treatment of pervasive developmental disorder. *Developmental and Behavioral Pediatrics, 7,* 73–76.

Flament, M. F., Rapoport, J. L., Berg, C. J., Sceery, W., Kilts, C., Mellstrom, B., & Linnoila, M. (1985). Clomipramine treatment of childhood obsessive–compulsive disorder. *Archives of General Psychiatry, 42,* 977–983.

Flaskerud, J. H., & Hu, L. T. (1994). Participation in and outcome of treatment for major depression among low-income Asian-Americans. *Psychiatry Research, 53,* 289–300.

Forness, S. R., Cantwell, D. P., Swanson, J. M., Hanna, G. L., & Youpa, D. (1991). Differential effects of stimulant medication on reading performance of boys with hyperactivity with and without conduct disorder. *Journal of Learning Disabilities, 24,* 304–310.

Forness, S. R., & Kavale, K. A. (1988). Psychopharmacological medication: A note on classroom effects. *Journal of Learning Disabilities, 21,* 144–147.

Fox, R. E., Schwelitz, F. D., & Barclay, A. G. (1992). A proposed curriculum for psychopharmacology training for professional psychologists. *Professional Psychology: Research and Practice, 23*, 216–219.

Frank, R. G. (1992). Prescription privileges for psychologists: Now is the time. *Physical Medicine and Rehabilitation: State of the Art Reviews, 6*, 577–583.

Freedman, J. E., Wirshing, W. C., Russell, A. T., Bray, M. P., & Unutzer, J. (1994). Absence status seizures during successful long-term clozapine treatment of an adolescent with schizophrenia. *Journal of Child and Adolescent Psychopharmacology, 4*, 53–62.

Gadow, K. D. (1981). Prevalence of drug treatment for hyperactivity and other childhood behavior disorders. In K. D. Gadow & J. Loney (Eds.), *Psychosocial aspects of drug treatment for hyperactivity* (pp. 13–76). Boulder, CO: Westview.

Gadow, K. D. (1982). Problems with students on medication. *Exceptional Children, 49*, 20–27.

Gadow, K. D. (1985). Prevalence and efficacy of stimulant drug use with mentally retarded children and youth. *Psychopharmacology Bulletin, 21*, 291–303.

Gadow, K. D. (1986). *Children on medication: Vol. I. Hyperactivity, learning disabilities, and mental retardation.* San Diego, CA: College-Hill Press.

Gadow, K. D. (1992). Pediatric psychopharmacotherapy: A review of recent research. *Journal of Child Psychology and Psychiatry and Allied Disciplines, 33*, 153–195.

Gadow, K. D. (1993a). A school-based medication evaluation program. In J. L. Matson (Ed.), *Handbook of hyperactivity in children* (1st ed., pp. 186–219). Needham Heights, MA: Allyn & Bacon.

Gadow, K. D. (1993b). Prevalence of drug therapy. In J. S. Werry & M. G. Aman (Eds.), *Practitioner's guide to psychoactive drugs for children and adolescents* (pp. 57–74). New York: Plenum.

Gadow, K. D. (in press). A school-based medication evaluation program. In J. Matson (Ed.), *Handbook of hyperactivity in children* (2nd ed.). Elmsford, NY: Pergamon Press.

Gadow, K. D., & Kalachnik, J. (1981). Prevalence and pattern of drug treatment for behavior disorders of TMR students. *American Journal of Mental Deficiencies, 85*, 588–595.

Gadow, K. D., & Nolan, E. E. (1993). Practical considerations in conducting school-based medication evaluations for children with hyperactivity. *Journal of Emotional and Behavioral Disorders, 1*, 118–126.

Gadow, K. D., Nolan, E. E., Paolicelli, L. M., & Sprafkin, J. (1991). A procedure for assessing the effects of methylphenidate on hyperactive children in public school settings. *Journal of Clinical Child Psychology, 20*, 268–276.

Gadow, K. D., Nolan, E. E., & Sverd, J. (1992). Methylphenidate in hyperactive boys with comorbid tic disorder: II. Short-term behavioral effects in school settings. *Journal of the American Academy of Child and Adolescent Psychiatry, 31*, 462–471.

Gadow, K. D., Nolan, E. E., Sverd, J., Sprafkin, J., & Paolicelli, L. M. (1990). Methylphenidate in aggressive–hyperactive boys: I. Effects on peer aggression in public school settings. *Journal of the American Academy of Child and Adolescent Psychiatry, 29*, 710–718.

Gadow, K. D., & Poling, A. (1988). *Pharmacotherapy and mental retardation*. San Diego, CA: College-Hill Press.

Gadow, K. D., Sverd, J., Sprafkin, J., Nolan, E. E., & Ezor, S. N. (1995). Efficacy of methylphenidate for attention-deficit hyperactivity disorder in children with tic disorder. *Archives of General Psychiatry, 52*, 444–455.

Gardos, G., Perenyi, A., Cole, J. O., Samu, I., & Kallos, M. (1983). Tardive dyskinesia: Changes after three years. *Journal of Clinical Psychopharmacology, 3*, 315–318.

Garfinkel, B. D., Wender, P. H., Sloman, L., & O'Neill, I. (1983). Tricyclic antidepressant and methylphenidate treatment of attention deficit disorder in children. *Journal of the American Academy of Child and Adolescent Psychiatry, 22*, 343–348.

Geller, B., Cooper, T. B., Graham, D. L., Fetner, H. H., Marsteller, F. A., & Wells, J. M. (1992). Pharmacokinetically designed double-blind placebo-controlled study of nortriptyline in 6- to 12-year-olds with major depressive disorder. *Journal of the American Academy of Child and Adolescent Psychiatry, 31*, 34–44.

Geller, B., Copper, T., Graham, D., Marsteller, F. A., & Bryant, D. M. (1989). Double-blind placebo-controlled study of nortriptyline in depressed adolescents using a "fixed plasma level" design. *Psychopharmacology Bulletin, 26*, 85–90.

Geller, B., Copper, T., McCombs, H., Graham, D., & Wells, J. (1989). Double-blind placebo-controlled study of nortriptyline in depressed children using a "fixed plasma level" design. *Psychopharmacology Bulletin, 26*, 101–108.

Geller, B., Fox, L. W., & Fletcher, M. (1993). Effect of tricyclic antidepressants on switching to mania and on the onset of bipolarity in depressed 6- to 12-year-olds. *Journal of the American Academy of Child and Adolescent Psychiatry, 32*, 43–50.

Geller, D. A., Biederman, J., Reed, E. D., Spencer, T., & Wilens, T. E. (1995). Similarities in response to fluoxetine in the treatment of children and adolescents with obsessive–compulsive disorder. *Journal of the American Academy of Child and Adolescent Psychiatry, 34*, 36–44.

Gillberg, C. (1991). The treatment of epilepsy in autism. *Journal of Autism and Developmental Disorders, 21*, 61–77.

Gittelman, R., Klein, D. F., & Feingold, I. (1983). Children with reading disorders—II: Effects of methylphenidate in combination with reading remediation. *Journal of Child Psychology and Psychiatry, 24*, 193–212.

Gittelman-Klein, R., & Klein, D. F. (1971). Controlled imipramine treatment of school phobia. *Archives of General Psychiatry, 25*, 204–207.

Gittelman-Klein, R., & Klein, D. F. (1973). School phobia: Diagnostic considerations in the light of imipramine effects. *Journal of Nervous and Mental Disease, 156*, 199–215.

Gittelman-Klein, R., Landa, B., Mattes, J. A., & Klein, D. F. (1988). Methylphenidate and growth in hyperactive children: A controlled withdrawal study. *Archives of General Psychiatry, 45*, 1127–1130.

Gittelman-Klein, R., & Mannuzza, S. (1988). Hyperactive boys almost grown up. III. Methylphenidate effects on ultimate height. *Archives of General Psychiatry, 45*, 1131–1134.

Golden, G. S. (1985). Tardive dyskinesia in Tourette syndrome. *Pediatric Neurology, 1,* 192–194.

Goodwin, F. K., & Jamison, K. R. (1990). *Manic–depressive illness.* London: Oxford University Press.

Gordon, C. T., Frazier, J. A., McKenna K., Giedd, J., Zametkin, A., Zahn, T., Hommer, D., Hong, W., Kaysen, D., & Albus, K. E. (1994). Childhood-onset schizophrenia: An NIMH study in progress. *Schizophrenia Bulletin, 20,* 697–712.

Gordon, M. (1983). *The Gordon Diagnostic System.* DeWitt, NY: Gordon Systems.

Goyette, C. H., Conners, C. K., & Ulrich, R. F. (1978). Normative data on Revised Conners' Parent and Teacher Rating Scales. *Journal of Abnormal Child Psychology, 6,* 221–236.

Graae, F., Milner, J., Rizzotto, L., & Klein, R. G. (1994). Clonazepam in childhood anxiety disorders. *Journal of the American Academy of Child and Adolescent Psychiatry, 33,* 372–376.

Gram, L. F., & Rafaelson, O. J. (1972). Lithium treatment of psychotic children and adolescents. *Acta Psychiatrica Scandinavica, 48,* 253–260.

Granger, D. A., Whalen, C., & Henker, B. (1993). Perceptions of methylphenidate effects on hyperactive children's peer interactions. *Journal of Abnormal Child Psychology, 21,* 535–549.

Green, W. H. (1995). *Child and adolescent clinical psychopharmacology* (2nd ed.). Baltimore: Williams & Wilkins.

Green, W. H., Padron-Gayol, M., Hardesty, A. S., & Bassiri, M. (1992). Schizophrenia with childhood onset: A phenomenological study of 38 cases. *Journal of the American Academy of Child and Adolescent Psychiatry, 31,* 968–976.

Greenberg, L. M., & Waldman, I. D. (1993). Developmental normative data on the Test of Variables of Attention (TOVA). *Journal of Child Psychology and Psychiatry and Allied Disciplines, 34,* 1019–1030.

Greenhill, L. L., Solomon, M., Pleak, R., & Ambrosini, P. (1985). Molindone hydrochloride treatment of hospitalized children with conduct disorder. *Journal of Clinical Psychiatry, 46,* 20–25.

Gualtieri, C. T., Quade, D., Hicks, R. E., Mayo, J. P., & Schroeder, S. R. (1988). Tardive dyskinesia and other clinical consequences of neuroleptic treatment in children and adolescents. *American Journal of Psychiatry, 141,* 20–23.

Gualtieri, C. T., Schroeder, S. R., Hicks, R. E., & Quade, D. (1986). Tardive dyskinesia in young mentally retarded individuals. *Archives of General Psychiatry, 43,* 335–340.

Gutkin, T. B. (1995). School psychology and health care: Moving service delivery into the twenty-first century. *School Psychology Quarterly, 10,* 236–246.

Guy, W. (1976a). Dosage Record and Treatment Emergent Symptoms Scale. In *ECDEU assessment manual for psychopharmacology* (rev.) (Publ. No. (ADM) 76–338, pp. 223–244). Washington, DC: U.S. Department of Health, Education and Human Welfare.

Guy, W. (1976b). Subjects Treatment Emergent Symptoms Scale. In *ECDEU assessment manual for psychopharmacology* (rev.) (Publ. No. (ADM) 76–338, pp. 347–350). Washington, DC: U.S. Department of Health, Education and Human Welfare.

Guy, W. (1976c). Abnormal Involuntary Movement Scale. In *ECDEU assessment manual for psychopharmacology* (rev.) (Publ. No. (ADM) 76–338 (pp. 534–537). Washington, DC: U.S. Department of Health, Education and Human Welfare.

Guy, W. (1976d). Physical and Neurological Examination for Soft Signs. *ECDEU assessment manual for psychopharmacology* (rev.) (Publ. No. (ADM) 76–338, pp. 383–406). Washington, DC: U.S. Department of Health, Education and Human Welfare.

Handen, B. J., Breaux, A. M., Gosling, A., Ploof, D. L., & Feldman, H. (1990). Efficacy of methylphenidate among mentally retarded children with attention deficit hyperactivity disorder. *Pediatrics, 86*, 922–930.

Hardman, J. G., Limbird, L. E., Molinoff, P. B., Ruddon, R. W., & Gilman, A. G. (Eds.). (1996). *Goodman & Gilman's: The pharmacological basis of therapeutics* (9th ed.). New York: McGraw-Hill.

Hauber, F.A., Bruininks, R. H., Hill, B. K., & Lakin, K. C. (1984). National census of residential facilities: A 1982 profile of facilities and residents. *American Journal of Mental Deficiency, 89*, 236–245.

Hauser, W. A., & Hesdorffer, D. C. (1990). *Epilepsy: Frequency, causes, and consequences.* New York: Demos.

Hazell, P., O'Connell, D., Heathcote, D., Robertson, J., & Henry, D. (1995). Efficacy of tricyclic drugs in treating child and adolescent depression: A meta-analysis. *British Medical Journal, 310*, 897–901.

Hechtman, L., & Weiss, G, (1983). Long-term outcome of hyperactive children. *American Journal of Orthopsychiatry, 53*, 532–541.

Hechtman, L., Weiss, G., & Perlman, T. (1984). Young adult outcome of hyperactive children who received long-term stimulant treatment. *Journal of the American Academy of Child and Adolescent Psychiatry, 23*, 261–269.

Hechtman, L., Weiss, G., Perlman, T., & Amsel, R. (1984). Hyperactives as young adults: Initial predictors of adult outcome. *Journal of the American Academy of Child and Adolescent Psychiatry, 23*, 250–260.

Henker, B., & Whalen, C. K. (1989). Hyperactivity and attention deficits. *American Psychologist, 44*, 216–233.

Henker, B., Whalen, C., Bugenthal, D. B., & Barker, C. (1981). Licit and illicit drug patterns in stimulant treated children and their peers. In K. D. Gadow & J. Loney (Eds.), *Psychosocial aspects of drug treatment for hyperactivity* (pp. 443–462). Boulder, CO: Westview.

Herjanic, B., & Reich, W. (1982). Development of a structured interview for children: Agreement between child and parent on individual symptoms. *Journal of Abnormal Child Psychology, 10*, 307–324.

Hill, B. K., Balow, E. A., & Bruininks, R. H. (1985). A national study of prescribed drugs in institutions and community residential facilities for mentally retarded people. *Psychopharmacology Bulletin, 21*, 279–284.

Hinshaw, S. P. (1991). Stimulant medication and the treatment of aggression in children with attention deficits. *Journal of Clinical Child Psychology, 20*, 301–312.

Hinshaw, S. P., Buhrmester, D., & Heller, R. (1989). Anger control in response to verbal provocation: Effects of stimulant medication for boys with ADHD. *Journal of Abnormal Child Psychology, 17*, 393–407.

Hinshaw, S. P., Henker, B., & Whalen, C. K. (1984). Self-control in hyperactive boys in anger-inducing situations: Effects of cognitive-behavioral training and of methylphenidate. *Journal of Abnormal Child Psychology, 12,* 55–77.

Hinshaw, S. P., Henker, B., Whalen, C., Erhardt, D., & Dunnington, R. E., Jr. (1989). Aggressive, prosocial, and nonsocial behavior in hyperactive boys: Dose effects of methylphenidate in naturalistic settings. *Journal of Consulting and Clinical Psychology, 57,* 636–643.

Holden, C. (1987). NIMH finds a case of "serious misconduct." *Science, 235,* 1566–1567.

Holowach, J., Thurstone, D. L., & O'Leary, J. (1972). Prognosis in childhood epilepsy: Follow-up study of 148 cases, in which therapy had been suspended after prolonged anticonvulsant control. *New England Journal of Medicine, 286,* 169–174.

Holttum, J. R., Lubetsky, M. J., & Eastman, L. E. (1994). Comprehensive management of trichotillomania in a young autistic girl. *Journal of the American Academy of Child and Adolescent Psychiatry, 33,* 577–581.

Hoy, E., Weiss, G., Minde, K., & Cohen, N. (1978). The hyperactive child at adolescence: Emotional, social, and cognitive functioning. *Journal of Abnormal Child Psychology, 6,* 311–324.

Hughes, C. W., Preskorn, S., Weller, E., Weller, R., Hassanein, R., & Tucker, S. (1990). The effect of concomitant disorders in childhood depression on predicting treatment response. *Psychopharmacology Bulletin, 26,* 235–238.

Humphries, T., Kinsbourne, M., & Swanson, J. (1978). Stimulant effects on cooperation and social interaction between hyperactive children and their mothers. *Journal of Child Psychology and Psychiatry, 19,* 13–22.

Hunt R. D., Capper, L., & O'Connell, P. (1990). Clonidine in child and adolescent psychiatry. *Journal of Child and Adolescent Psychopharmacology, 1,* 87–102.

Hunt, R. D., Minderaa, R. B., & Cohen, D. J. (1985). Clonidine benefits children with attention deficit disorder and hyperactivity: Report of a double-blind placebo-crossover therapeutic trial. *Journal of the American Academy of Child Psychiatry, 24,* 617–629.

Ialongo, N. S., Lopez, M., Horn, W. F., Pascoe, J. M., & Greenberg, G. (1994). Effects of psychostimulant medication on self-perceptions of competence, control, and mood in children with attention deficit hyperactivity disorder. *Journal of Clinical Child Psychology, 23,* 161–173.

Jacobs, B. L. (1994). Serotonin, motor activity, and depression-related disorders. *American Scientist, 82,* 456–463.

Jacobvitz, D., Sroufe, L. A., Stewart, M., & Leffert, N. (1990). Treatment of attentional and hyperactivity problems in children with sympathomimetic drugs: A comprehensive review. *Journal of the American Academy of Child and Adolescent Psychiatry, 29,* 677–688.

Jaffee, J. H. (1985). Drug addiction and drug abuse. In A. G. Gilman, L. S. Goodman, T. W. Rall, & F. Murad (Eds.), *The pharmacological basis of therapeutics* (pp. 532–581). New York: Macmillan.

Jain, U., Birmaher, B., Garcia, M., Al-Shabbout, M., & Ryan, N. (1992). Fluoxetine in children and adolescents with mood disorders: A chart review of efficacy and adverse effects. *Journal of Child and Adolescent Psychopharmacology, 2,* 259–265.

Jastak, S., & Wilkinson, G. S. (1990). *Wide Range Achievement Test–Revised*. Wilmington, DE: Jastak Associates.

Johnston, C., & Fine, S. (1993). Methods of evaluating methylphenidate in children with attention-deficit hyperactivity disorder: Acceptability, satisfaction, and compliance. *Journal of Pediatric Psychology, 18*, 717–730.

Joshi, P. T., Capozzoli, J. A., & Coyle, J. T. (1988). Low-dose neuroleptic therapy for children with childhood-onset pervasive developmental disorder. *American Journal of Psychiatry, 145*, 335–338.

Kagan, J. (1965). Reflection–impulsivity: The generality and dynamics of conceptual tempo. *Journal of Abnormal Psychology, 71*, 17–24.

Kandel, E. R., Schwartz, J. H., & Jessell, T. M. (1991). *Principles of neural science* (3rd ed.). New York: Elsevier.

Kashani, J., Shekim, W., & Reid, J. (1984). Amitriptyline in children with minor depressive disorder: A double-blind crossover pilot study. *Journal of the American Academy of Child and Adolescent Psychiatry, 23*, 348–351.

Kaslow, N., Brown, R. T., & Mee, L. (1994). Contemporary cognitive-behavioral models for childhood depression. In W. M. Reynolds & H. F. Johnston (Eds.), *Handbook of depression in children and adolescents* (pp, 97–121). New York: Plenum.

Kaslow, N. J., Rehm, L. P., & Siegel, A. W. (1984). Social–cognitive and cognitive correlates of depression in children. *Journal of American Child Psychology, 12*, 605–620.

Kasten, E. F., Coury, D. L., & Heron, T. E. (1992). Educators' knowledge and attitudes regarding stimulants in the treatment of attention deficit hyperactivity disorder. *Journal of Developmental and Behavioral Pediatrics, 13*, 215–219.

Kauffman, R. E., Smith-Wright, D., Reese, C. A., Simpson, R., & Fowler, J. (1981). Medication compliance in hyperactive children. *Pediatric Psychopharmacology, 1*, 231–237.

Kazdin, A. E. (1980). Acceptability of alternative treatments for deviant behavior. *Journal of Applied Behavior Analysis, 13*, 259–273.

Kazdin, A. E. (1981). Acceptability of child treatment techniques: The influence of treatment efficacy and adverse side effects. *Behavior Therapy, 12*, 493–506.

Kazdin, A. E. (1984). Acceptability of aversive procedures and medication as treatment alternatives for deviant child behavior. *Journal of Abnormal Child Psychology, 12*, 289–302.

Kazdin, A. E., French, N. H., & Sherick, R. A. (1981). Acceptability of alternative treatments for children: Evaluations by inpatient children, parents, and staff. *Journal of Consulting and Clinical Psychology, 49*, 900–907.

Keith, R. W., & Engineer, P. (1991). Effects of methylphenidate on the auditory processing of children with attention deficit–hyperactivity disorder. *Journal of Learning Disabilities, 24*, 630–636.

Keller, M. B., Lavori, P. W., Beardslee, W. R., Wunder, J., & Ryan, N. (1991). Depression in children and adolescents: New data on "undertreatment" and a literature review on the efficacy of available treatments. *Journal of Affective Disorders, 21*, 163–171.

Kilbey, M. M., Brown, R. T., Coursey, R. D., Eisdorser, C., France, C., Johnson, D. L., Kirschner, N. M., Martin, J., Macure, C., Morris, J., Sammons,

M. T., Strickland, T. L., Thompson, T. I., & Vuchinich, R. E. (1995). *Final report of the BEA Working Group to develop a level 1 curriculum for psychopharmacology education and training.* Washington, DC: American Psychological Association.

Kilbey, M. M., Brown, R. T., Coursey, R. D., Eisdorser, C., France, C., Johnson, D. L., Kirschner, N. M., Martin, J., Macure, C., Morris, J., Sammons, M. T., Strickland, T. L., Thompson, T. I., & Vuchinich, R. E. (1996). *Final report of the BEA Working Group to develop a level 2 curriculum for psychopharmacology education and training.* Washington, DC: American Psychological Association.

King, R. A., Riddle, M. A., Chappell, P. B., Hardin, M. T., Anderson, G. M., Lombroso, P., & Scahill, L. (1991). Emergence of self-destructive phenomena in children and adolescents during fluoxetine treatment. *Journal of the American Academy of Child and Adolescent Psychiatry, 30,* 179–186.

Klee, S., & Garfinkel, B. (1984). Identification of depression in children and adolescents: The role of the dexamethasone suppression test. *Journal of the American Academy of Child and Adolescent Psychiatry, 23,* 410–415.

Klein, R. G. (1988). Childhood anxiety disorders. In C. J. Kestenbaum & D. T. Williams (Eds.), *Clinical assessment of children and adolescents: A biopsychosocial approach* (pp. 722–742). New York: New York University Press.

Klein, R. G., & Koplewicz, H. S. (1990). *Desipramine treatment in adolescent depression.* Paper presented at the Child Depression Consortium meeting, Pittsburgh, PA.

Klein, R. G., Koplewicz, H. S., & Kanner, A. (1992). Imipramine treatment of children with separation anxiety disorder. *Journal of the American Academy of Child and Adolescent Psychiatry, 31,* 21–28.

Klein, R. G., & Last, C. G. (1989). *Anxiety disorders in children.* Newbury Park, CA: Sage.

Klorman, R., Brumaghim, J. T., Fitzpatrick, P. A., & Borgstedt, A. D. (1990). Clinical effects of a controlled trial of methylphenidate on adolescents with attention deficit disorder. *Journal of the American Academy of Child and Adolescent Psychiatry, 29,* 702–709.

Klorman, R., Brumaghim, J. T., Fitzpatrick, P. A., & Borgstedt, A. D., & Strauss, J. (1994). Clinical and cognitive effects of methylphenidate on children with attention deficit disorder as a function of aggression/oppositionality and age. *Journal of Abnormal Psychology, 103,* 206–221.

Klorman, R., Brumaghim, J. T., Salzman, L. F., Strauss, J., Gorgstedt, A. D., McBride, M. C., & Loeb, S. (1988). Effects of methylphenidate on attention-deficit hyperactivity disorder with and without aggressive/noncompliant features. *Journal of Abnormal Psychology, 97,* 413–422.

Kovacs, M. (1985). The Children's Depression Inventory (CDI). *Psychopharmacology Bulletin, 21,* 995–998.

Kovacs, M., Feinberg, T. L., Crouse-Novak, M. A., Paulauskas, S. L., & Finkelstein, R. (1984). Depressive disorders in childhood: I. A longitudinal prospective study of characteristics and recovery. *Archives of General Psychiatry, 41,* 229–237.

Kowatch, R. A., Suppes, T., Gilfillan, S. K., Fuentes, R. M., Grannemann, B. D., Emslie, G. J. (1995). Clozapine treatment of children and adolescents with bipolar disorder and schizophrenia: A clinical case series. *Journal of Child and Adolescent Psychopharmacology, 5*, 241–253.(ch3, 4)

Kraft, I. A., Ardall, C., Duffy, J. H., Hart, J. T., & Pearce, P. A. (1965). A clinical study of chlordiazepoxide used in psychiatric disorders in children. *International Journal of Neuropsychiatry, 1*, 433–437.

Krakowski, A. J. (1963). Chlordiazepoxide in treatment of children with emotional disturbances. *New York State Journal of Medicine, 63*, 3388–3392.

Kramer, A., & Feiguine, R. (1981). Clinical effects of amitriptyline in adolescent depression. *Journal of the American Academy of Child and Adolescent Psychiatry, 20*, 636–644.

Kranzler, H. R., & Liebowitz, N. R. (1988). Anxiety and deptession in substance abuse: Clinical implications. *Medical Clinics of North America, 72*, 867–885.

Kratochowill, T. R. (1994). Psychopharmacology for children and adolescents: Commentary on current issues and future challenges. *School Psychology Quarterly, 9*, 53–59.

Krener, P. K., & Mancina, R. A. (1994). Informed consent or informed coercion? Decision-making in pediatric psychopharmacology. *Journal of Child and Adolescent Psychopharmacology, 4*, 183–200.

Kruesi, M. J. P., Rapoport, J. L., Hamburger, S., Hibbs, E., Potter, W. Z., Lenane, M., & Brown, G. L. (1990). Cerebrospinal fluid metabolites, aggression, and impulsivity in disruptive behavior disorders of children and adolescents. *Archives of General Psychiatry, 47*, 419–426.

Kubiszyn, T., & Carlson, C. I. (1995). School psychologists' attitudes toward an expanded health care role: psychopharmacology and prescription privileges. *School Psychology Quarterly, 10*, 247–270.

Kupietz, S. S., Winsberg, B. G., Richardson, E., Maitinsky, S., & Mendell, N. (1988). Effects of methylphenidate dosage in hyperactive reading-disabled children: I. Behavior and cognitive performance effects. *Journal of the American Academy of Child and Adolescent Psychiatry, 27*, 70–77.

Kutcher, S. P., Boulos, C., Ward, B., Marton, P., Simeon, J., Ferguson, H. B., Szalai, J., Katic, M., Roberts, N., Dubois, C., & Reed, K. (1994). Response to desipramine treatment in adolescent depression: A fixed-dose, placebo-controlled trial. *Journal of the American Academy of Child and Adolescent Psychiatry, 33*, 686–694.(ch3, 5)

Kutcher, S. P., & MacKenzie, S. (1988). Successful clonazepam treatment of adolescents with panic disorder [Letter to the editor]. *Journal of Clinical Psychopharmacology, 8*, 299–301.

Kutcher, S. P., Reiter, S., Gardner, D. M., & Klein, R. G. (1992). The pharmacotherapy of anxiety disorders in children and adolescents. *Psychiatric Clinics of North America, 15*, 41–68.

Kye, C. H., Waterman, G. S., Ryan, N. D., Birmaher, B., Williamson, D. E., Iyengar, S., & Dachille, S. (1996). A randomized, controlled trial of amitriptyline in the acute treatment of adolescent major depression. *Journal of the American Academy of Child and Adolescent Psychiatry, 35*, 1139–1144.

LaGreca, A., & Schulman, W. (1995). Adherence to prescribed medical regimes. In M. Roberts (Ed.), *Handbook of pediatric psychology* (2nd ed., pp. 55–83). New York: Guilford Press.

Landau, S., & Moore, L. A. (1991). Social skill deficits in children with attention-deficit hyperactivity disorder. *School Psychology Review, 20,* 235–251.

Landgraf, J. M., Abetz, L., & Ware, J. E., Jr. (1997). *The Child Health Questionnaire (CHQ): A user's manual.* Boston: The Health Institute, New England Medical Center.

Latz, S. R., & McCracken, J. T. (1992). Neuroleptic malignant syndrome in children and adolescents: Two case reports and a warning. *Journal of Child and Adolescent Psychopharmacology, 2,* 123–129.

Leonard, H. L., Meyer, M. C., Swedo, S. E., Richter, D., Hamburger, S. D., Allen, A. J., Rapoport, J. L., & Tucker, E. (1995). Electrocardiographic changes during desipramine and clomipramine treatment in children and adolescents. *Journal of the American Academy of Child and Adolescent Psychiatry, 34,* 1460–1468.

Leonard, H. L., Swedo, S. E., & Lenane, M. C. (1993). A 2- to 7-year follow-up study of 54 obsessive–compulsive children and adolescents. *Archives of General Psychiatry, 50,* 429–439.

Leonard, H. L., Swedo, S. E., Rapoport, J. L, Koby, E. V., Lenane, M. C., Cheslow, D. L., & Hamburger, S. D. (1989). Treatment of obsessive–compulsive disorder with clomipramine and desipramine in children and adolescents: A double-blind crossover comparison. *Archives of General Psychiatry, 46,* 1088–1092.

Licamele, W. L., & Goldberg, R. L. (1989). The concurrent use of lithium and methylphenidate in a child. *Journal of the American Academy of Child and Adolescent Psychiatry, 28,* 785–787.

Liebowitz, M. R., Hollander, E., Fairbanks, J., & Campeas, R. (1990). Fluoxetine for adolescents with obsessive–compulsive disorder. *American Journal of Psychiatry, 147,* 370–371.

Liu, C., Robin, A. L., Brenner, A., & Eastman, J. (1991). Social acceptability of methylphenidate and behavior modification for treating attention deficit hyperactivity disorder. *Pediatrics, 88,* 560–565.

Loney, J., Kramer, J., & Milich, R. (1981). The hyperactive child grows up: Predictors of symptoms, delinquency, and achievement at follow-up. In K. Gadow & J. Loney (Eds.), *Psychosocial aspects of drug treatment for hyperactivity* (pp. 381–415). Boulder, CO: Westview.

Lucas, A. R., & Pasley, F. C. (1969). Psychoactive drugs in the treatment of emotionally disturbed children: Haloperidol and diazepam. *Comprehensive Psychiatry, 10,* 376–386.

Malone, M. A., Kershner, J. R., & Seigel, L. (1988). The effects of methylphenidate on levels of processing and laterality in children with attention deficit disorder. *Journal of Abnormal Child Psychology, 16,* 379–395.

Malone, M. A., & Swanson, J. M. (1993). Effects of methylphenidate on impulsive responding in children with attention deficit hyperactivity disorder. *Journal of Child Neurology, 8,* 157–163.

Malyn, A., Jenson, W. R., & Clark, E. (1993, March). *Myths and realities about ADHD: A comprehensive survey of school psychologists and teachers about causes and treatments.* Paper presented at the annual convention of the National Association of School Psychologists, Washington, DC.

Matier, K., Halperin, J. M., Sharma, V., Newcorn, J. H., & Sathaye, N. (1992).

Methylphenidate response in aggressive and nonaggressive ADHD children: Distinctions on laboratory measures of symptoms. *Journal of the American Academy of Child and Adolescent Psychiatry, 31,* 219–225.

McClellan, J., & Werry, J. (1994). Practice parameters for the assessment and treatment of children and adolescents with schizophrenia. *Journal of the American Academy of Child and Adolescent Psychiatry, 33,* 616–635.

Meiselas, K. D., Spencer, E. K., Oberfield, R., Peselow, E.D., Angrist, B., & Campbell, M. (1989). Differentiation of stereotypies from neuroleptic-related dyskinesias in autistic children. *Journal of Clinical Psychopharmacology, 9,* 207–209.

Meltzer, H. Y. (1992). Dimensions of outcome with clozapine. *British Journal of Psychiatry, 160* (Suppl. 17), 46–53.

Mendelson, J. H., Johnson, N. E., Stewart, M. A. (1971). Hyperactive children as teenagers: A follow-up study. *Journal of Nervous and Mental Disease, 153,* 273–279.

Meyerhoff, J. L., & Snyder, S. H. (1973). Gilles de la Tourette's disease and minimal brain dysfunction: Amphetamine isomers reveal catecholamine correlates in an affected patient. *Psychopharmacologia, 29,* 211–220.

Miczek, K. A. (1987). The psychopharmacology of aggression. In L. L. Iversen, S. D. Iversen, & S. H. Snyder (Eds.), *Handbook of psychopharmacology: New directions in behavioral pharmacology* (pp. 183–328). New York: Plenum.

Milich, R. (1994). The response of children with ADHD to failure: If at first you don't succeed, do you try, try, again? *School Psychology Review, 23,* 11–28.

Milich, R., Carlson, A. L., Pelham, W. E., & Licht, B. G. (1991). Effects of methylphenidate on the persistence of ADHD boys following failure experiences. *Journal of Abnormal Child Psychology, 19,* 519–536.

Milich, R., & Kramer, J. (1985). Reflections on impulsivity: An empirical investigation of impulsivity as a construct. In K. Gadow & I. Bialer (Eds.), *Advances in learning and behavioral disabilities* (Vol. 3, pp. 117–150). Greenwich, CT: JAI Press.

Milich, R., Licht, B. G., Murphy, D. A., & Pelham, W. E. (1989). Attention-deficit hyperactivity disordered boys' evaluations of attributions for task performance on medication versus placebo. *Journal of Abnormal Child Psychology, 98,* 280–284.

Minde, K., Weiss, G., & Mendelson, N. (1972). A 5-year follow-up study of 91 hyperactive school children. *Journal of the American Academy of Child Psychiatry, 11,* 595–610.

Mitchell, W. G., Zhou, Y., Chavez, J. M., & Guzman, B. L. (1993). Effects of antiepileptic drugs on reaction time, attention, and impulsivity in children. *Pediatrics, 91,* 101–105.

Mittle, V. F., & Robin, A. (1987). Acceptability of alternative interventions for parent–adolescent conflict. *Behavioral Assessment, 9,* 417–428.

Mozes, T., Toren, P., Chernauzan, N., Mester, R., Yoran-Hegesh, R., Blumensohn, R., & Weizman, A. (1994). Clozapine treatment in very early onset schizophrenia. *Journal of the American Academy of Child and Adolescent Psychiatry, 33,* 65–70.

Murphy, D. A., Pelham, W. E., & Lange, A. R. (1992). Aggression in boys with attention deficit–hyperactivity disorder: Methylphenidate effects on naturalistically observed aggression, response to provocation, and social information processing. *Journal of Abnormal Child Psychology, 20,* 451–466.

National Institute of Mental Health. (1985). Rating scales and assessment instruments for use in pediatric psychopharmacology research. *Psychopharmacology Bulletin, 21*[Special issue 4].

Nolan, E. E., & Gadow, K. D. (1994). Relation between ratings and observations of stimulant drug response in hyperactive children. *Journal of Clinical Child Psychology, 23,* 78–90.

Nolan, E. E., & Gadow, K. D., & Sverd, J. (1994). Observations and ratings of tics in school settings. *Journal of Abnormal Child Pstchology, 22,* 579–593.

Nolan, E. E., Sverd, J., Gadow, K. D., Sprafkin, J., & Ezor, S. N. (1996). Associated psychopathology in children with both ADHD and chronic tic disorder. *Journal of the American Academy of Child and Adolescent Psychiatry, 35,* 1622–1630.

Nolte, R., Wetzel, B., & Brugmann, G. (1979). Effects of phenytoin and primidone monotherapy on mental performance in children. In S. I. Johannessen, P. L. Morselli, & C. E. Pippenger (Eds.), *Antiepileptic therapy: Advances in drug monitoring* (pp. 81–86). New York: Raven Press.

Nurcombe, B., & Partlett, D. F. (1994). *Child mental health and the law.* New York: Free Press.

O'Dougherty, M., Wright, F. S., Cox, S., & Walson, P. (1987). Carbamazepine plasma concentration relationship to cognitive impairment. *Archives of Neurology, 44,* 863–867.

Padgett, R., & Lipman, E. (1989). Use of neuroleptics after an episode of neuroleptic malignant syndrome. *Canadian Journal of Psychiatry, 34,* 323–325.

Paulson, G. W., Rizvi, C. A., & Crane, G. E. (1975). Tardive dyskinesia as a possible sequel of long-term therapy with the phenothiazines. *Clinical Pediatrics, 14,* 953–955.

Paxton, J. W., & Dragunow, M. (1993). Pharmacology. In J. S. Werry & M. G. Aman (Eds.), *Practitioner's guide to psychoactive drugs for children and adolescents* (pp. 23–55). New York: Plenum.

Peacock, L., Solgaard, T., Lubin, H., & Gerlach, J. (1996). Clozapine versus typical antipsychotics: A retrospective and prospective study of extrapyramidal side effects. *Psychopharmacology, 124,* 188–196.

Pelham, W. (1986). The effects of psychostimulant drugs on learning and academic achievement in children with attention-deficit disorders and learning disabilities. In J. Torgesen & B. Wong (Eds.), *Psychological and educational perspectives on learning disabilities* (pp. 259–295). New York: Academic Press.

Pelham, W. E. (1993). Pharmacotherapy for children with attention-deficit hyperactivity disorder. *School Psychology Review, 22,* 199–227.

Pelham, W. E., & Bender, M. E. (1982). Peer relationships in hyperactive children: Description and treatment. In K. Gadow & I. Bailer (Eds.), *Advances in learning and behavioral disabilities* (Vol. 1, pp. 365–436). Greenwich, CT: JAI Press.

Pelham, W. E., Bender, M. E., Caddell, J., Booth, S., & Moorer, S. H. (1985). Methylphenidate and children with attention deficit disorder. *Archives of General Psychiatry, 42,* 948–952.

Pelham, W. E., & Hoza, J. (1987). Behavioral assessment of psychostimulant effects on ADD children in a summer day treatment program. In R. Prinz (Ed.), *Advances in behavioral assessment of children and families* (Vol. 3, pp. 3–34). Greenwich, CT: JAI Press.

Pelham, W. E., Murphy, D. A., Vannatta, K., Milich, R., Licht, B. G., Gnagy, E. M., Greenslade, K. E., Greiner, A. R., & Vodde-Hamilton, M. (1992). Methylphenidate and attributions in boys with attention-deficit hyperactivity disorder. *Journal of Consulting and Clinical Psychology, 60*, 282–292.

Pelham, W. E., Vallano, G., Hoza, B., Greiner, A. R., & Gnagy, E. M. (1992). *Methylphenidate dose effects on ADHD children: Individual differences across children and domains.* Unpublished manuscript, University of Pittsburgh, Pittsburgh, PA.

Pelham, W. E., Vodde-Hamilton, M., Murphy, D. A., Greenstein, J., & Vallano, G. (1990). The effects of methylphenidate on ADHD adolescents in recreational, peer group, and classroom settings. *Journal of Clinical Child Psychology, 20*, 293–300.

Peloquin, L. J., & Klorman, R. (1986). Effects of methylphenidate on normal children's mood, event-related potentials, and performance in memory scanning and vigilance. *Journal of Abnormal Psychology, 95*, 88–98.

Perl, R. (1992, November 8). Overdosing on Ritalin. *The Atlanta Journal/Constitution*, pp. 7–9.

Petti, T. A., Fish, B., Shapiro, T., Cohen, I. L., & Campbell, M. (1982). Effects of chlordiazepoxide in disturbed children: A pilot study. *Journal of Clinical Psychopharmacology, 2*, 270–273.

Petti, T., & Law, W. (1982). Imipramine treatment of depressed children: A double-blind pilot study. *Journal of Clinical Psychopharmacology, 2*, 107–110.

Pfefferbaum, G., Overall, J. E., Boren, H. A., Frankel, L. S., Sullivan, M. R., & Johnson, K. (1987). Alprazolam in the treatment of anticipatory and acute situational anxiety in children with cancer. *Journal of the American Academy of Child and Adolescent Psychiatry, 26*, 532–535.

Piccinelli, M., Pini, S., Bellantuono, C., & Wilkinson, G. (1995). Efficacy of drug treatment in obsessive–compulsive disorder: A meta-analytic review. *British Journal of Psychiatry, 166*, 424–443.

Piotrowski, C., & Keller, J. W. (1996, March). *Do psychologists want to be retrained for prescription privileges?* Paper presented at the annual meeting of the Southeastern Psychological Association, Norfolk, VA.

Platt, J. E., Campbell, M., Green, W. H., & Grega, D. M. (1984). Cognitive effects of lithium carbonate and haloperidol in treatment-resistant aggressive children. *Archives of General Psychiatry, 41*, 657–662.

Pleak, R. R., Birmaher, B., Gavrilescu, A., Abichandani, C., & Williams, D. T. (1988). Mania and neuropsychiatric excitation following carbamazepine. *Journal of the American Academy of Child and Adolescent Psychiatry, 27*, 500–503.

Pliszka, S. R. (1987). Tricyclic antidepressants in the treatment of children with deficit disorder. *Journal of the American Academy of Child and Adolescent Psychiatry, 26*, 127–132.

Pliszka, S. R. (1991). Antidepressants in the treatment of child and adolescent psychopathology. *Journal of Clinical Child Psychology, 20*, 313–320.

Pliszka, S. R., McCracken, J. T., & Maas, J. W. (1996). Catecholamines in attention-deficit hyperactivity disorder: Current perspectives. *Journal of the American Academy of Child and Adolescent Psychiatry, 35,* 264–272.

Poling, A., Gadow, K. D., & Cleary, J. (1991a). *Drug therapy for behavior disorders: An introduction.* New York: Pergamon.(

Poling, A., Gadow, K. D., & Cleary, J. (1991b). Neuroleptics. In *Drug therapy for behavior disorders: An introduction* (pp. 49–73). New York: Pergamon Press.

Polizos, P., Englehardt, D. M., Hoffman, S. P., & Waizer, J. (1973). Neurological consequences of psychotropic drug withdrawal in schizophrenic children. *Journal of Autism and Childhood Schizophrenia, 3,* 247–253.

Pool, D., Bloom, W., Mielke, D. H., Roniger, J. J., & Gallant, D. M. (1976). A controlled evaluation of loxitane in seventy-five schizophrenic adolescents. *Current Therapy Research, 19,* 99–104.

Pope, H. G., Hudson, J. I., Jonas, J. M., & Yurgelun-Todd, D. (1983). Bulimia treated with imipramine: A placebo-controlled, double-blind study. *American Journal of Psychiatry, 140,* 554–558.

Porrino, L. J., Rapoport, J. L., Behar, D., Ismond, D. R., & Bunney, W. E., Jr. (1983). A naturalistic assessment of the motor activity of hyperactive boys. II. Stimulant drug effects. *Archives of General Psychiatry, 40,* 688–693.

Porteus, S. D. (1967). *The Porteus Maze test manual.* London: George C. Harrap.

Power, T. J., Hess, L. E., & Bennett, D. S. (1995). The acceptability of interventions for attention deficit disorder among elementary and middle school teachers. *Developmental and Behavioral Pediatrics, 16,* 238–243.

Preskorn, S. H., & Jerkovich, G. (1990). Central nervous system toxicity of tricyclic antidepressants: Phenomenology, course, risk factors, and role of therapeutic drug monitoring. *Journal of Clinical Psychopharmacology, 10,* 88–95.

Preskorn, S. H., Jerkovich, G. S., Beber, J. H., & Widener, P. (1989). Therapeutic drug monitoring of tricyclic antidepressants: A standard of care issue. *Psychopharmacology Bulletin, 25,* 281–284.

Preskorn, S. H., Weller, E. B., Hughes, C. W., Weller, R. A., & Bolte, K. (1987). Depression in prepubertal children: Dexamethasone nonsuppression predicts differential response to imipramine vs. placebo. *Psychopharmacology Bulletin, 23,* 450–453.

Puig-Antich, J., Perel, J. M., Lupatkin, W., Chambers, W. J., Tabrizi, M. A., King, J., Goetz, R., Davies, M., & Stiller, R. L. (1987). Imipramine in prepubertal major depressive disorders. *Archives of General Psychiatry, 44,* 81–89.

Rapoport, J., L. Abramson, A., Alexander, D., & Lott, I. (1971). Playroom observations on hyperactive children on medication. *Journal of the American Academy of Child Psychiatry, 10,* 524–534.

Rapoport, J. L., Quinn, P. O., Bradbard, G., Riddle, D., & Brooks, E. (1974). Imipramine and methylphenidate treatments of hyperactive boys: A double-blind comparison. *Archives of General Psychiatry, 30,* 789–793.

Rapport, M. D., Carlson, G. A., Kelly, K. L, & Petaki, C. (1993). Methylphenidate and desipramine in hospitalized children: I. Separate and combined effects on cognitive function. *Journal of the American Academy of Child and Adolescent Psychiatry, 32,* 333–342.

Rapport, M. D., Denney, C., DuPaul, G. J., & Gardner, M. J. (1994). Attention deficit disorder and methylphenidate: Normalization rates, clinical effectiveness, and response prediction in 76 children. *Journal of the American Academy of Child and Adolescent Psychiatry, 33*, 882–893.

Rapport, M. D., DuPaul, G. J., Stoner, G., & Jones, J. T. (1986). Comparing classroom and clinic measures of attention deficit disorder: Differential, idiosyncratic, and dose-response effects of methylphenidate. *Journal of Consulting and Clinical Psychology, 54*, 334–341.

Rapport, M. D., & Kelly, K. L. (1991). Psychostimulant effects on learning and cognitive function in children with attention deficit hyperactivity disorder: Findings and implications. In J. L. Matson (Ed.), *Hyperactivity in children: A handbook*. New York: Pergamon Press.

Rapport, M. D., Quinn, S. O., DuPaul, G. J., Quinn, E. P., & Kelly, K. L. (1989). Attention deficit disorder with hyperactivity and methylphenidate: The effects of dose and mastery level on children's learning performance. *Journal of Abnormal Child Psychology, 17*, 669–689.

Realmuto, G. M., August, G. J., & Garfinkel, B. D. (1989). Clinical effects of buspirone in autistic children. *Journal of Clinical Psychopharmacology, 9*, 122–125.

Realmuto, G. M., Erickson, W. D., Yellin, A., Hopwood, J. H., & Greenberg, L. M. (1984). Clinical comparison of thiothixene and thioridazine in schizophrenic adolescents. *American Journal of Psychiatry, 141*, 440–442.

Reid, M. K., & Borkowski, J. G. (1984). Effects of methylphenidate (Ritalin) on information processing in hyperactive children. *Journal of Abnormal Child Psychology, 12*, 169–186.

Reynolds, C. R., & Paget, K. D. (1983). National normative and reliability data for the Revised Children's Manifest Anxiety Scale. *School Psychology Review, 12*, 324–336.

Richardson, E., Kupietz, S. A., Winsberg, B. G., Maitinsky, S., & Mendell, N. (1988). Effects of methylphenidate dosage in hyperactive reading-disabled children: II. Reading achievement. *Journal of the American Academy of Child and Adolescent Psychiatry, 27*, 78–87.

Richardson, M. A., Haugland, G., & Craig, T. J. (1991). Neuroleptic use, Parkinsonian symptoms, tardive dyskinesia, and associated factors in child and adolescent psychiatric patients. *American Journal of Psychiatry, 148*, 1322–1328.

Richman, N., Douglas, J., Hunt, H., Lansdown, R., & Levere, R. (1985). Behavioral methods in the treatment of sleep disorders: A pilot study. *Journal of Child Psychology and Psychiatry, 26*, 581–598.

Richters, J. E., Arnold, L. E., Jensen, P. S., Abikoff, H., Conners, C. K., Greenhill, L., Hechtman, L., Hinshaw, S. P., Pelham, W. E., & Swanson, J. M. (1995). NIMH collaborative multisite multimodal treatment study of children with ADHD: I. Background and rationale. *Journal of the American Academy of Child and Adolescent Psychiatry, 34*, 987–1000.

Rickels, K., & Schweizer, E. (1995). Long-term treatment of anxiety disorders. *Psychopharmacology Bulletin, 31*, 115–123.

Riddle, K. D., & Rapoport, J. L. (1976). A 2-year follow-up of 72 hyperactive boys. *Journal of Nervous and Mental Disease, 162*, 126–134.

Riddle, M. A., Geller, B., & Ryan, N. (1993). Another sudden death in a child treated with desipramine. *Journal of the American Academy of Child and Adolescent Psychiatry, 32*, 792–797.

Riddle, M. A., Hardin, M. T., King, R., Scahill, L., & Woolston, J. L. (1990). Fluoxetine treatment of children and adolescents with Tourette's and obsessive compulsive disorders: Preliminary clinical experience. *Journal of the American Academy of Child and Adolescent Psychiatry, 29,* 45–48.

Riddle, M. A., King, R. A., Hardin, M. T., Scahill, L., Ort, S. I., Chappell, P., Rasmusson, A., & Leckman, J. F. (1990). Behavioral side effects of fluoxetine in children and adolescents. *Journal of Child and Adolescent Psychopharmacology, 1,* 193–198.

Riddle, M. A., Lynch, K. A., Scahill, L., DeVries, A., Cohen, D. J., & Leckman, J. F. (1995). Methylphenidate discontinuation and reinitiation during long-term treatment of children with Tourette's disorder and attention-deficit hyperactivity disorder: A pilot study. *Journal of Child and Adolescent Psychopharmacology, 5,* 205–214.

Riddle, M. A., Scahill, L., King, R. A., Hardin, M. T., Anderson, G. M., Ort, S. I., Smith, J. C., Leckman, J. F., & Cohen, D. J. (1992). Double-blind, crossover trial of fluoxetine and placebo in children and adolescents with obsessive-compulsive disorder. *Journal of the American Academy of Child and Adolescent Psychiatry, 31,* 1062–1069.

Rimland, B. (1988). Controversies in the treatment of autistic children: Vitamin and drug therapy. *Journal of Child Neurology, 3* (Suppl.), 68–72.

Roberts, M. C. (1986). *Pediatric psychology: Psychological interventions and strategies for pediatric problems.* New York: Pergamon Press.

Romanczyk, R. G. (1986). Self-injurious behavior: Conceptualization, assessment, and treatment. In K. D. Gadow (Ed.), *Advances in learning and behavioral disabilities* (Vol. 5, pp. 29–56). Greenwich, CT: JAI Press.

Rosenberg, D. R., Holttum, J., & Gershon, S. (1994). *Textbook of pharmacotherapy for child and adolescent psychiatric disorders.* New York: Brunner Mazel.

Rosenberg, D. R., Johnson, K., & Sahl, R. (1992). Evolving mania in an adolescent treated with low-dose fluoxetine. *Journal of Child and Adolescent Psychopharmacology, 2,* 299–306.

Ross, D. C., & Piggott, L. R. (1993). Clonazepam for OCD [Letter to the editor]. *Journal of the American Academy of Child and Adolescent Psychiatry, 32,* 470–471.

Rudorfer, M. V., & Robins, E. (1982). Amitriptyline overdose: Clinical effects on tricyclic antidepressant plasma levels. *Journal of Clinical Psychiatry, 43,* 457–460.

Safer, D. J., & Allen, R. P. (1973). Factors influencing the suppressant effects of two stimulant drugs on the growth of hyperactive children. *Pediatrics, 51,* 660–667.

Safer, D. J., Allen, R. P., & Barr, E. (1972). Depression of growth in hyperactive children on stimulant drugs. *New England Journal of Medicine, 287,* 217–220.

Safer, D. J., & Krager, J. M. (1988). A survey of medication treatment for hyperactive/inattentive students. *Journal of the American Medical Association, 260,* 2256–2258.

Safer, D. J., & Krager, J. M. (1989). Hyperactivity and inattentiveness: School assessment of stimulant treatment. *Clinical Pediatrics, 28,* 216–221.

Safer, D. J., Zito, J. M., & Pine, E. M. (1996). Increased methylphenidate usage for attention deficit disorder in the 1990s. *Pediatrics, 98,* 1084–1088.

Sallee, F., Stiller, R., & Perel, J. (1992). Pharmacodynamics of pemoline in attention deficit disorder with hyperactivity. *Journal of the American Academy of Child and Adolescent Psychiatry, 31*, 244–251.

Sammons, M. T. (1994). Prescription privileges and psychology: A reply to Adams and Bieliauskas. *Journal of Clinical Psychology in Medical Settings, 1*, 199–207.

Satterfield, J. H., Hoppe, C. M., & Schill, A. M. (1982). A prospective study of delinquency in 110 adolescent boys with attention deficit disorder and 88 normal adolescent boys. *American Journal of Psychiatry, 139*, 797–798.

Satterfield, J. H., Satterfield, B. T., & Cantwell, D. P. (1981). Three-year multimodal treatment study of 100 hyperactive boys. *Behavioral Pediatrics, 98*, 650–655.

Sattler, J. M. (1986). Assessment of behavior by observational methods. *Assessment of children* (3rd ed., pp. 472–530). San Diego, CA: Jerome M. Sattler.

Schachar, R., Hoppe, C., & Schell, A. (1987). Changes in family function and relationships in children who respond to methylphenidate. *Journal of the American Academy of Child and Adolescent Psychiatry, 26*, 728–732.

Schachar, R., & Tannock, R. (1993). Childhood hyperactivity and psychostimulants: A review of extended treatment studies. *Journal of Child and Adolescent Psychopharmacology, 3*, 81–91.

Schachar, R., Taylor, E., Wieselberg, M., Thorley, G., & Rutter, M. (1987). Changes in family function and relationships in children who respond to methylphenidate. *Journal of the American Academy of Child and Adolescent Psychiatry, 26*, 728–732.

Schain, R. J., Ward, J. W., & Guthrie, D. (1977). Carbamazepine as an anticonvulsant in children. *Neurology, 27*, 476–480.

Schleifer, M., Weiss, G., Cohen, N., Elman, M., Crejic, H., & Kruger, E. (1975). Hyperactivity in preschoolers and the effect of methylphenidate. *American Journal of Orthopsychiatry, 45*, 33–50.

Schmidt, M. H., Trott, G. E., Blanz, B., & Nissen, G. (1990). Clozapine medication in adolescents. In C. N. Stefania, A. D. Rabavilas, & C. R. Soldatos (Eds.), Psychiatry: A world perspective. Proceedings of the VIII World Congress of Psychiatry, Amsterdam. *Excerpta Medica, 1*, 1100–1104.

Schouten, R., & Duckworth, K. S. (1993). Medicolegal and ethical issues in the pharmacologic treatment of children. In J. S. Werry & M. G. Aman (Eds.), *Practitioner's guide to psychoactive drugs for children and adolescents*. New York: Plenum.

Schroeder, S. R., & Gualtieri, C. T. (1985). Behavioral interactions induced by chronic neuroleptic therapy in persons with mental retardation. *Psychopharmacology Bulletin, 21*, 310–315.

Sebrechts, M. M., Shaywitz, S. E., Shaywitz, B. A., Jatlow, P., Anderson, G. M., & Cohen, D. J. (1986). Components of attention, methylphenidate dosage, and blood levels in children with attention deficit disorder. *Pediatrics, 77*, 222–228.

Shapiro, A. K., & Shapiro, E. (1984). Controlled study of pimozide versus placebo in Tourette's syndrome. *Journal of the American Academy of Child and Adolescent Psychiatry, 23*, 161–173.

Shapiro, A. K., Shapiro, E., & Eisenkraft, G. J. (1983). Treatment of Gilles de la

Tourette syndrome with pimozide. *American Journal of Psychiatry, 140,* 1183–1186.

Shapiro, E., Shapiro, A. K., Young, J. G., & Feinberg, T. E. (1988). *Gilles de la Tourette syndrome.* New York: Raven Press.

Shaywitz, S. E., & Shaywitz, B. A. (1994). Learning disabilities and attention disorders. In K. Swaiman (Ed.), *Pediatric neurology* (pp. 1119–1151). Baltimore: Mosby.

Shelton, T., & Barkley, R. A. (1995). The assessment and treatment of attention deficit hyperactivity disorder in children. In M. Roberts (Ed.), *Handbook of pediatric psychology* (2nd ed., pp. 633–754). New York: Guilford Press.

Sigelman, C. K., & Shorokey, J. J. (1986). Effects of treatments and their outcomes on peer perceptions of a hyperactive child. *Journal of Abnormal Child Psychology, 14,* 397–410.

Silva, R. R., Magee, H. J., & Friedhoff, A. J. (1993). Persistent tardive dyskinesia and other neuroleptic-related dyskinesias in Tourette's disorder. *Journal of Child and Adolescent Psychopharmacology, 3,* 137–144.

Silverstein, F. S., Parrish, M. A., & Johnston, M. V. (1982). Adverse behavioral reactions in children treated with carbamazepine (Tegretol). *Journal of Pediatrics, 101,* 785–787.

Simeon, J. G. (1991). Buspirone effects in adolescent psychiatric disorders. *European Neuropsychopharmacology, 1,* 421.

Simeon, J. G., Dinicola, V. F., Ferguson, H. B., & Copping, W. (1990). Adolescent depression: A placebo-controlled fluoxetine treatment study and follow-up. *Progress in Neuro-psychopharmacological and Biological Psychiatry, 14,* 791–795.

Simeon, J. G., & Ferguson, H. B. (1987). Alprazolam effects in children with anxiety disorders. *Canadian Journal of Psychiatry, 32,* 570–574.

Simeon, J. G., Ferguson, H. B., & Fleet, J. V. W. (1986). Bupropion effects in attention deficit and conduct disorder. *Canadian Journal of Psychiatry, 31,* 581–585.

Simeon, J. G., Ferguson, H. B., Knott, V., Roberts, N., Gauthier, B., Dubois, C., & Wiggins, D. (1992). Clinical, cognitive, and neurophysiological effects of alprazolam in children and adolescents with overanxious and avoidant disorders. *Journal of the American Academy of Child and Adolescent Psychiatry, 31,* 29–33.

Simeon, J. G., Knott, V. J., DuBois, C., Wiggins, D., Geraets, I., Thatte, S., & Miller, W. (1994). Buspirone therapy of mixed anxiety disorders in children and adolescents: A pilot study. *Journal of Child and Adolescent Psychopharmacology, 4,* 159–170.

Singh, N. N., Epstein, M. H., Luebke, J., & Singh, Y. N. (1990). Psychopharmacological intervention. I: Teacher perceptions of psychotropic medication for students with serious emotional disturbance. *Journal of Special Education, 24,* 283–295.

Sleator, E. K. (1985). Measurement of compliance. *Psychopharmacology Bulletin, 21,* 1089–1093.

Slimmer, L. W., & Brown, R. T. (1985). Parents' decision-making process in medication administration for control of hyperactivity. *Journal of School Health, 55,* 221–225.

Smith, P. F., & Darlington, C. L. (1996). *Clinical psychopharmacology: A primer.* Mahwah, NJ: Erlbaum.

Smyer, M. A., Balster, R. L., Egli, D., Johnson, D. L., Kilbey, M. M., Leith, N. J., & Puente, A. E. (1992, July). *Report of the ad hoc task force on psychopharmacology of the American Psychological Association*. Washington, DC: American Psychological Association.

Smyer, M. A., Balster, R. L., Egli, D., Johnson, D. L., Kilbey, M. M., Leith, N. J., & Puente, A. E. (1993). Summary of the report of the ad hoc task force on psychopharmacology of the American Psychological Association. *Professional Psychology: Research and Practice, 24,* 394–403.

Solanto, M. V. (1991). Dosage effects of Ritalin on cognition. In L. L. Greenhill & B. B. Osmon (Eds.), *Ritalin: Theory and patient management* (pp. 233–246). New York: Mary Ann Liebert.

Solanto, M. V., & Wender, E. K. (1989). Does methylphenidate constrict cognitive functioning? *Journal of the American Academy of Child and Adolescent Psychiatry, 28,* 897–902.

Spencer, E. K., Kafantaris, V., Padron-Gayol, M., Rosenberg, C. R., & Campbell, M. (1992). Haloperidol in schizophrenic children: Early findings from a study in progress. *Psychopharmacology Bulletin, 28,* 183–186.

Spencer, T., Biederman, J., Kerman, K., Steingard, R., & Wilens, T. (1993). Desipramine treatment of children with attention-deficit hyperactivity disorder and tic disorder or Tourette's syndrome. *Journal of the American Academy of Child and Adolescent Psychiatry, 32,* 354–360.

Spencer, T., Biederman, J., Wilens, T., Harding, M., O'Donnell, D., & Griffin, S. (1996). Pharmacotherapy of attention-deficit hyperactivity disorder across the life cycle. *Journal of the American Academy of Child and Adolescent Psychiatry, 35,* 409–432.

Sprague, R. L., & Newell, K. M. (1987). Toward a movement control perspective of tardive dyskinesia. In H. Y. Meltzer (Ed.), *Psychopharmacology: The third generation of progress* (pp. 1233–1238). New York: Raven Press.

Sprague, R., & Sleator, E. (1977). Methylphenidate in hyperkinetic children: Differences in dose effects on learning and social behavior. *Science, 198,* 1274–1276.

Sroufe, L. A., & Stewart, M. A. (1973). Treating problem children with stimulant drugs. *New England Journal of Medicine, 289,* 407–413.

Stefl, M. E., Bornstein, R. A., & Hammond, L. (1988). *The 1987 Ohio Tourette survey*. Milford: Tourette Syndrome Association of Ohio.

Steingard, R. J., DeMaso, D. R., Goldman, S. J., Shorrock, K. L., & Bucci, J. P. (1995). Current perspectives on the pharmacotherapy of depressive disorders in children and adolescents. *Harvard Review of Psychiatry, 2,* 313–326.

Steingard, R. J., Khan, A., Gonzalez, A., & Herzog, D. B. (1992). Neuroleptic malignant syndrome: Review of experience with children and adolescents. *Journal of Child and Adolescent Psychopharmacology, 2,* 183–198.

Stephens, R. S., Pelham, W. E., & Skinner, R. (1984). State-dependent and main effects of methylphenidate and pemoline on paired-associate learning and spelling in hyperactive children *Journal of Consulting and Clinical Psychology, 52,* 104–113.

Stokes, P. E. (1993). Fluoxetine: A five-year review. *Clinical Therapeutics, 15,* 216–243.

Stores, G., Williams, P. L., Styles, E., & Zaiwalla, Z. (1992). Psychological effects of sodium valproate and carbamazepine in epilepsy. *Archives of Disabilities of Children, 67,* 1330–1337.

Streiner, D. L., & Norman, G. R. (1995). *Health measurement scales: A practical guide to their development and use* (2nd ed). Oxford, England: Oxford University Press.

Strickland, T. L., Lin, K. M., Fu, P., Anderson, D., & Zheng, Y. (1995). Comparison of lithium ratio between African-American and Caucasian bipolar patients. *Biological Psychiatry, 37,* 325–330.

Sulzbacher, S. I. (1973). Psychotropic medication with children: An evaluation of procedural biases in results of reported studies. *Pediatrics, 51,* 513–517.

Summers, J. A., & Caplan, P. J. (1987). Lay people's attitudes toward drug treatment for behavioral control depend on which disorder and which drug. *Clinical Pediatrics, 26,* 258–263.

Sverd, J., Gadow, K. D., Nolan, E. E., Sprafkin, J., & Ezor, S. N. (1992). Methylphenidate in hyperactive boys with comorbid tic disorder: I. Clinic evaluations. In T. N. Chase, A. J. Friedhoff, & D. J. Cohen (Eds.), *Advances in neurology: Vol. 58. Tourette syndrome 2: A decade of progress.* (pp. 271–281). New York: Raven Press.

Sverd, J., Gadow, K. D., & Paolicelli, L. M. (1989). Methylphenidate treatment of attention-deficit hyperactivity disorder in boys with Tourette syndrome. *Journal of the American Academy of Child and Adolescent Psychiatry, 28,* 574–579.

Swanson, J. M. (1985). Measures of cognitive functioning appropriate for use in pediatric psychopharmacology studies. *Psychopharmacology Bulletin, 21,* 887–892.

Swanson, J. M. (1989). Paired-associate learning in the assessment of ADD-H children. In L. M. Bloomingdale & J. Swanson (Eds.), *Attention deficit disorder: Current concepts and emerging trends in attentional and behavioral disorders of childhood* (pp. 87–123). New York: Pergamon Press.

Swedo, S. E., & Leonard, H. L. (1994). Childhood movement disorders and obsessive compulsive disorder. *Journal of Clinical Psychiatry, 55,* 32–37.

Tannock, R., Ickowicz, A., & Schachar, R. (1995). Differential effects of methylphenidate on working memory in ADHD children with and without comorbid anxiety. *Journal of the American Academy of Child and Adolescent Psychiatry, 34,* 886–896.

Tannock, R., Schachar, R. J., Carr, R. P., & Logan, G. D. (1989). Dose–response effects of methylphenidate on academic performance and overt behavior in hyperactive children. *Pediatrics, 84,* 648–657.

Tarnowski, K. J., Gavaghan, M. P., & Wisniewski, J. J. (1989). Acceptability of interventions for pediatric pain management. *Journal of Pediatric Psychology, 14,* 463–472.

Tarnowski, K. J., Kelly, P. A., & Mendlowitz, D. R. (1987). Acceptability of behavioral pediatric interventions. *Journal of Consulting and Clinical Psychology, 55,* 435–436.

Tarnowski, K. J., Simonian, S. J., Bekeny, P., & Park, A. (1992). Acceptability of interventions for childhood depression. *Behavior Modification, 16,* 103–117.

Task Force on Late Effects of Antipsychotic Drugs. (1980). Tardive dyskinesia:

Summary of a task force report of the American Psychiatric Association. *American Journal of Psychiatry, 137,* 1163–1172.

Taylor, E. (1994). Physical treatments. In M. Rutter, E. Taylor, & L. Hersov (Eds.), *Child and adolescent psychiatry: Modern approaches* (pp. 880–899). Melbourne, Australia: Blackwell.

Taylor, S. E., & Brown, J. D. (1988). Illusion and well-being: A social-psychological perspective on mental health. *Psychological Bulletin, 103,* 193–210.

Teicher, M. H., Glod, C., & Cole, J. O. (1990). Emergence of intense suicidal preoccupation during fluoxetine treatment. *American Journal of Psychiatry, 147,* 207–210.

Todt, H. (1984). The late prognosis of epilepsy in childhood: Results of a prospective follow-up study. *Epilepsia, 25,* 137–144.

Trimble, M. R., & Corbett, J. (1980). Anticonvulsant drugs and cognitive function. In J. A. Wada & J. K. Penry (Eds.), *Advances in epileptology: The Xth epilepsy international symposium* (pp. 113–120). New York: Raven Press.

Turkkan, J. S. (1995). Antihypertensives: Pharmacotherapy side effects in women: Psychopharmacology from a feminist perspective. *Women and Therapy, 16* [Special Issue], 49–71.

Urman, R., Ickowicz, A., Fulford, P., & Tannock, R. (1995). An exaggerated cardiovascular response to methylphenidate in ADHD children with anxiety. *Journal of Child and Adolescent Psychopharmacology, 5,* 29–37.

Varanka, T. M., Weller, R. A., Weller, E. B., & Fristad, M. A. (1988). Lithium treatment of manic episodes with psychotic features in prepubertal children. *American Journal of Psychiatry, 145,* 1557–1559.

Varley, C. K., & Trupin, E. (1982). Double-blind administration of methylphenidate to mentally retarded children with attention deficit disorder: A preliminary study. *American Journal of Mental Deficiency, 86,* 560–566.

Viesselman, J. O., Yaylayan, S., Weller, E. B., & Weller, R. A. (1993). Antidysthymic drugs (antidepressants and antimanics). In J. S. Werry & M. G. Aman (Eds.), *Practitioner's guide to psychoactive drugs for children and adolescents* (pp. 239–268). New York: Plenum.

Vining, E. P., Mellitis, E. D., Dorsen, M. M., Cataldo, M. F., Quaskey, S. A., Spielberg, S. P., & Freeman, J. M. (1987). Psychologic and behavioral effects of antiepileptic drugs in children: A double blind comparison between phenobarbital and valproic acid. *Pediatrics, 80,* 165–174.

Vitiello, B., Hill, J. L., & Elia, J. (1991). P.R.N. medication in child psychiatric patients: A pilot placebo-controlled study. *Journal of Clinical Psychiatry, 52,* 499–501.

Voeller, K. S., Marcus, B. A., & Lewis, M. H. (1993). Multiple estimates of dopaminergic function in ADHD children [abstract]. *Biological Psychiatry, 33,* 110A.

Volkmar, F. R., & Nelson, D. S. (1990). Seizure disorders in autism. *Journal of the American Academy of Child and Adolescent Psychiatry, 29,* 127–129.

Vyse, S. A., & Rapport, M. D. (1989). The effects of methylphenidate on learning in children with ADHD: The stimulus-equivalence paradigm. *Journal of Consulting and Clinical Psychology, 57,* 425–435.

Waizer, J., Hoffman, S. P., Pulizos, P., & Engelhardt, D. M. (1974). Outpatient treatment of hyperactive school children with imipramine. *American Journal of Psychiatry, 131,* 587–591.

Waters, B. G. H. (1990). Psychopharmacology of the psychiatric disorders of childhood and adolescence. *Medical Journal of Australia, 152,* 32–39.

Weiss, G. (1983). Long-term outcome: Findings, concepts, and practical implications. In M. Rutter (Ed.), *Developmental neuropsychiatry* (pp. 422–449). New York: Guilford Press.

Weiss, G. (1985). Followup studies on outcome of hyperactive children. *Psychopharmacology Bulletin, 21,* 169–177.

Weiss, G. & Hechtman, L. T. (1986). *Hyperactive children grown up.* New York: Guilford Press.

Weiss, G., Hechtman, L., Milroy, T., & Perlman, T. (1985). Psychiatric status of hyperactives as adults: A controlled prospective 15-year follow-up of 63 hyperactive children. *Journal of the American Academy of Child Psychiatry, 24,* 211–220.

Weiss, G., Kruger, E., Danielson, V., & Elman, M. (1975). Effects of long-term treatment of hyperactive children with methylphenidate. *Canadian Medical Association Journal, 112,* 159–165.

Werry, J. S. (1978). Measures in pediatric psychopharmacology. In J. S. Werry (Ed.), *Pediatric psychopharmacology: The use of behavior modifying drugs in children* (pp. 29–78). New York: Brunner/Mazel.

Werry, J. S., & Aman, M. G. (1975). Methylphenidate and haloperidol in children: Effects on attention, memory, and activity. *Archives of General Psychiatry, 32,* 790–795.

Werry, J. S., & Aman, M. G. (1993a). Anxiolytics, sedatives, and miscellaneous drugs. In J. S. Werry & M. G. Aman (Eds.), *Practitioner's guide to psychoactive drugs for children and adolescents* (pp. 391–415). New York: Plenum.

Werry, J. S., & Aman, M. G. (Eds.). (1993b). *Practitioner's guide to psychoactive drugs for children and adolescents.* New York: Plenum.

Werry, J. S., Aman, M. G., & Lampen, E. (1975). Haloperidol and methylphenidate in hyperactive children. *Acta Paedopsychiatrica, 42,* 26–40.

Werry, J. S., Dowrick, P. W., Lampen, E. L., & Vamos, M. J. (1975). Imipramine in enuresis: Psychological and physiological effects. *Journal of Child Psychology, Psychiatry, and Allied Disciplines, 16,* 289–299.

Werry, J. S., Weiss, G., Douglas, V., & Martin, J. (1966). Studies on the hyperactive child: III. The effect of chlorpromazine upon behavior and learning ability. *Journal of the American Academy of Child and Adolescent Psychiatry, 5,* 292–312.

Westermeyer, J. (1987). Cultural factors in clinical assessment. *Journal of Consulting and Clinical Psychology, 55,* 471–478.

Whalen, C. K., Collins, B. E., Henker, B., Alkus, S. R., Adams, D., & Stapp, J. (1978). Behavior observations of hyperactive children and methylphenidate (Ritalin) effects in systematically structured classroom environments: Now you see them, now you don't. *Journal of Pediatric Psychology, 3,* 177–187.

Whalen, C. K., & Henker, B. (1976). Psychostimulants and children: A review and analysis. *Psychological Bulletin, 83,* 1113–1130.

Whalen, C. K., & Henker, B. (1991a). Social impact of stimulant treatment for hyperactive children. *Journal of Learning Disabilities, 24,* 231–241.

Whalen, C. K., & Henker, B. (1991b). Therapies for hyperactive children: Comparison, combinations, and compromises. *Journal of Consulting and Clinical Psychology, 59,* 126–137.

Whalen, C. K., & Henker, B. (in press). Attention-deficit/hyperactivity disorders. In T. H. Ollendick & M. Hersen (Eds.), *Handbook of child psychopathology* (3rd ed.). New York: Plenum.

Whalen, C. K., Henker, B., Buhrmester, D., Hinshaw, S. P., Huber, A., & Laski, K. (1989). Does stimulant medication improve the peer status of hyperactive children? *Journal of Consulting and Clinical Psychology, 57,* 545–549.

Whalen, C. K., Henker, B., Castro, B., & Granger, D. (1987). Peer perceptions of hyperactivity and medication effects. *Child Development, 58,* 816–828.

Whalen, C. K., Henker, B., Collins, B. E., Finck, D., & Dotemoto, S. (1979). A social ecology of hyperactive boys: Medication effects in structured classroom environments. *Journal of Applied Behavior Analysis, 12,* 65–81.

Whalen, C. K., Henker, B., Collins, B. E., McAuliffe, S., & Vaux, A. (1979). Peer interaction in a structured communication task: Comparisons of normal and hyperactive boys and of methylphenidate (Ritalin) and placebo effects. *Child Development, 50,* 388–401.

Whalen, C. K., Henker, B., & Dotemoto, S. (1980). Methylphenidate and hyperactivity: Effects on teacher behaviors. *Science, 208,* 1280–1282.

Whalen, C. K., Henker, B., & Dotemoto, S. (1981). Teacher response to the methylphenidate (Ritalin) versus placebo status of hyperactive boys in the classroom. *Child Development, 52,* 1005–1014.

Whalen, C. K., Henker, B., & Finck, D. (1981). Medication effects in the classroom: Three naturalistic indicators. *Journal of Abnormal Child Psychology, 9,* 419–433.

Whalen, C. K., Henker, B., Hinshaw, S. P., Heller, T., & Huber-Dressler, A. (1991). Messages of medication: Effects of actual versus informed medication status on hyperactive boys' expectancies and self-evaluations. *Journal of Consulting and Clinical Psychology, 59,* 602–606.

Whalen, C. K., Henker, B., Swanson, J. M., Granger, D., Kliewer, W., & Spencer, J. (1987). Natural social behaviors in hyperactive children: Dose effects of methylphenidate. *Journal of Consulting and Clinical Psychology, 55,* 187–193.

Whitaker, A., & Rao, U. (1992). Neuroleptics in pediatric psychiatry. In D. Shaffer (Ed.), *The psychiatric clinics of North America* (Vol. 15, pp. 243–276). Philadelphia: Saunders.

Wiener, J. M. (1996). *Diagnosis and psychopharmacology of childhood and adolescent disorders* (2nd ed.). New York: Wiley.

Wilkison, P. C., Kircher, J. C., McMahon, W., & Sloan, H. N. (1995). Effects of methylphenidate on reward strength in boys with attention-deficit hyperactivity disorder. *Journal of the American Academy of Child and Adolescent Psychiatry, 34,* 897–901.

Wolraich, M. L., Lindgren, S., Stromquist, A., Milich, R., Davis, C., & Watson, D. (1990). Stimulant medication use by primary care physicians in the treatment of attention deficit hyperactivity disorder. *Pediatrics, 86,* 95–101.

Woodcock, R. W. (1989). *Woodcock–Johnson Psycho-educational Battery–Revised.* Allen, TX: DLM Teaching Resources.

Wright, H. H., Cuccaro, M. L., Leonhardt, T. V., Kendall, D. F., & Anderson, J. H. (1995). Case study: Fluoxetine in the multimodal treatment of a preschool child with selective mutism. *Journal of the American Academy of Child and Adolescent Psychiatry, 34,* 857–862.

Yang, Y. Y. (1985). Prophylactic efficacy of lithium and its effective plasma levels in Chinese bipolar patients. *Acta Psychiatrica Scandinavica, 71,* 171–175.

Zametkin, A. J., Nordahl, T. E., & Gross, M. (1990). Cerebral glucose metabolism in adults with hyperactivity of childhood onset. *New England Journal of Medicine, 323,* 1361–1366.

Zametkin, A. J., & Yamada, E. M. (1993). Monitoring and measuring drug effects: I. Physical effects. In J. S. Werry & M. G. Aman (Eds.), *Practitioner's guide to psychoactive drugs for children and adolescents* (pp. 75–97). New York: Plenum.

Zeiner, P. (1995). Body growth and cardiovascular function after extended treatment (1.75 years) with methylphenidate in boys with attention-deficit hyperactivity disorder. *Journal of Child and Adolescent Psychopharmacology, 5,* 129–138.

Zhang, Y. A., Reviriego, J., Lou, Y. Q., Sjoqvist, F., & Bertilsson, L. (1990). Diazepam metabolism in native Chinese poor and extensive hydroxylators of S-mephenytoin: Interethnic differences in comparison with white subjects. *Clinical Pharmacology and Therapeutics, 48,* 496–502.

Zwier, K. J., & Rao, U. (1994). Buspirone use in an adolescent with social phobia and mixed personality disorder (cluster A type). *Journal of the American Academy of Child and Adolescent Psychiatry, 33,* 1007–1011.

Index

♦